Healthcare Simulation in Nursing Practice

Editor

PENNI I. WATTS

NURSING CLINICS
OF NORTH AMERICA

www.nursing.theclinics.com

Consulting Editor
BENJAMIN SMALLHEER

September 2024 • Volume 59 • Number 3

ELSEVIER

1600 John F. Kennedy Boulevard • Suite 1800 • Philadelphia, Pennsylvania, 19103-2899

http://www.theclinics.com

NURSING CLINICS OF NORTH AMERICA Volume 59, Number 3
September 2024 ISSN 0029-6465, ISBN-13: 978-0-443-13111-0

Editor: Kerry Holland
Developmental Editor: Malvika Shah

Nursing Clinics of North America (ISSN 0029-6465) is published quarterly by Elsevier Inc., 360 Park Avenue South, New York, NY 10010-1710. Months of issue are March, June, September, and December. Periodicals postage paid at New York, NY and additional mailing offices. Subscription price per year is, $168.00 (US individuals), $275.00 (international individuals), $231.00 (Canadian individuals), $100.00 (US and Canadian students), and $135.00 (international students). For institutional access pricing please contact Customer Service via the contact information below. To receive student/resident rate, orders must be accompanied by name of affiliated institution, date of term, and the signature of program/residency coordinator on institution letterhead. Orders will be billed at individual rate until proof of status is received. Foreign air speed delivery is included in all *Clinics* subscription prices. All prices are subject to change without notice. Orders, claims, and journal inquiries: Please visit our Support Hub page https://service.elsevier.com for assistance.

Nursing Clinics of North America is covered in *EMBASE/Excerpta Medica, MEDLINE/PubMed (Index Medicus), Social Sciences Citation Index, Current Contents, ASCA, Cumulative Index to Nursing, RNdex Top 100,* and Allied Health Literature and International Nursing Index (INI).

Contributors

CONSULTING EDITOR

BENJAMIN SMALLHEER, PhD, RN, ACNP-BC, FNP-BC, CCRN, CNE, FAANP
Assistant Dean, Master of Science in Nursing Program, Associate Professor, Duke University School of Nursing, Durham, North Carolina

EDITOR

PENNI I. WATTS, PhD, CHSE-A, RN, FNAP, ANEF, FSSH, FAAN
Assistant Director, UAB Office of Interprofessional Curriculum, Associate Professor, Associate Dean for Technology and Innovation, Acute, Chronic and Continuing Care, The University of Alabama at Birmingham School of Nursing, Birmingham, Alabama, USA

AUTHORS

SABRINA BEROZ, DNP, RN, ANEF, CHSE-A
Professor Emerita, Montgomery College, Consultant, National League for Nursing, Gaithersburg, Maryland, USA

FARA BOWLER, DNP, APRN, CHSE
Associate Professor, College of Nursing, University of Colorado, Aurora, Colorado, USA

JENNIFER DALE-TAM, RN, MSN, CNCC(c), CCSNE, CHSE
Corporate Simulation Nurse Educator, The Ottawa Hospital, Ottawa, Ontario, Canada

DESIREE A. DÍAZ, PhD, FNP-BC, CNE, CHSE-A, ANEF, FSSH, FAAN
Professor, Department of Nursing Practice, College of Nursing, Academic Health Sciences Center, University of Central Florida, Orlando, Florida, USA

CRYSTEL L. FARINA, PhD, RN, CNE, CHSE
Associate Dean of BSN Programs, Department of Nursing, George Washington University School of Nursing, Ashburn, Virginia, USA

MARY K. FEY, PhD, RN, CHSE-A, ANEF, FAAN
Associate Director, Applied Learning for Performance and Safety, Principal Faculty, Center for Medical Simulation, Boston, Massachusetts, USA

DARLA GRUBEN, EdD(c), MSN, CHSE, CNE
Assistant Professor, College of Nursing, The University of North Texas Health Science Center, Fort Worth, Texas, USA

BETH FENTRESS HALLMARK, PhD, RN, MSN, CHSE-A, ANEF
Associate Professor, Inman College of Nursing, Director of Education Simulation Center, Belmont Simulation Center, Belmont University, Nashville, Tennessee, USA

ELIZABETH HORSLEY, RN, MSMS, CHSE, CCSNE
Formerly, Director of Simulation, The Brooklyn Hospital Center, Brooklyn, New York; Currently, Vineland, Ontario, Canada

BRANDON KYLE JOHNSON, PHD, RN, CHSE, ANEF
Executive Director, TTUHSC Simulation Program, Associate Professor, TTUHSC School of Nursing, Texas Tech University Health Sciences Center, Lubbock, Texas, USA

JESSICA L. KAMERER, EDD, MSN, RNC-NIC
Director, Corporate Programs and Lifetime Learning, Assistant Director, Center for Innovative Teaching, Associate Faculty, Nursing, Robert Morris University, Moon Township, Pennsylvania, USA

JARED M. KUTZIN, DNP, MS, MPH, RN, FSSH, FAAN
Associate Professor, Emergency Medicine and Medical Education, Icahn School of Medicine at Mount Sinai, Senior Director, Simulation, Teaching, and Research Center, The Mount Sinai Hospital, New York, New York, USA

KATHEE LAFFOON, MSN/Ed, RN, PHN, RNC-OB, CHSE
Professional Development Specialist, Center for Learning and Innovation, Scripps Health, San Diego, California, USA

HUMBERTO LÓPEZ CASTILLO, MD, PhD, CPH, CMI-Spanish
Assistant Professor, Department of Health Sciences, College of Health Professions and Sciences, Academic Health Sciences Center, Assistant Professor, Department of Population Health Sciences, College of Medicine, Academic Health Sciences Center, University of Central Florida, Orlando, Florida, USA

YUTING LIN, PhD, MSN, RN
Assistant Professor, Seattle University-College of Nursing, Seattle, Washington, USA

CONNIE M. LOPEZ, MSN, CNS, CPHRM, CHSE-A, FSSH
Clinical Practice Consultant, Quality and Safety Improvement Consultant, Perinatal Patient Safety, Risk and Patient Safety, Northern California Region, Kaiser Permanente, Oakland, California, USA

PATRICK LUNA, MSN, RN, CEN
Senior Instructor, College of Nursing, University of Colorado, Aurora, Colorado, USA

VALERIE C. MARTÍNEZ, DNP, APRN, CPNP-PC, PMHS
Clinical Assistant Professor, Department of Nursing Practice, College of Nursing, Academic Health Sciences Center, University of Central Florida, Orlando, Florida, USA

DONNA S. McDERMOTT, PhD, RN, CHSE-A
Professor of Nursing, Associate Dean of Simulation, University of South Florida College of Nursing, Tampa, Florida, USA

CARRIE WESTMORELAND MILLER, PHD, RN, CNE, CHSE, IBCLC, FAAN
Associate Professor, Montana State University-Mark and Robyn Jones College of Nursing, Billings, Montana, USA

JASLINE MORENO, MSN, RN, CHSE-A, CNE
Faculty Lead, Maryland Clinical Resource Consortium, Montgomery College, Takoma Park, Maryland, USA

KATE J. MORSE, PhD, MSN, RN, CHSE, ACNP-Ret, FAAN
Assistant Dean, Experiential Learning and Innovation, Associate Clinical Professor or Nursing, College of Nursing and Health Professions, Drexel University, Philadelphia, Pennsylvania, USA

KELLY ROSSLER, PhD, RN, CHSE, CNE
Associate Professor, Louise Herrington School of Nursing, Baylor University, Dallas, Texas, USA

MARY SCHAFER, MSN, RN, CHSE
Lecturer, East Tennessee State University, Johnson City, Tennessee, USA

TONYA SCHNEIDEREITH, PhD, MBA, CRNP, PPCNP-BC, CPNP-AC, CNE, CHSE-A, ANEF, FSSH, FAAN
Chief Operating Officer of SIMPL Simulation, LLC, Brooklandville, Maryland, USA

SAMANTHA SMELTZER, DNP, RN, CHSE
Director of Simulation and Integrated Simulation Operations, Orbis Education, Indianapolis, Indiana, USA

TEDRA SMITH, DNP, CPNP-PC, CNE, CHSE
Associate Professor, Assistant Dean for Graduate Clinical Education - MSN, Director, Pediatric Partnerships, The University of Alabama at Birmingham School of Nursing, Birmingham, Alabama, USA

TAMMY SPENCER, DNP, RN, CNE, ACNS-BC
Associate Professor, College of Nursing, University of Colorado, Aurora, Colorado, USA

BECKY SUTTLE, DNP, BS, CRNP, AGACNP-BC
Assistant Professor, Director, Nurse Practitioner Pathways-DNP, The University of Alabama at Birmingham School of Nursing, Birmingham, Alabama, USA

JENNIFER TAYLOR, MSN, RN, NPD-BC, CCRN-K
Baylor Scott & White Health, Baylor University Medical Center, Center for Nursing Education and Research, Dallas, Texas, USA

CARMAN TURKELSON, DNP, RN, CCRN-K, CHSE-A
Associate Professor of Nursing and Director of School of Nursing, Center for Simulation and Clinical Innovation, School of Nursing, University of Michigan-Flint, Flint, Michigan, USA

ELIZABETH WELLS-BEEDE, PhD, RN, C-EFM, CHSE-A, CNE, ACUE, FAAN
Senior Associate Dean, College of Nursing, The University of North Texas Health Science Center, Fort Worth, Texas, USA

TRACIE WHITE, DNP, ACNP-BC, CRNFA, CNOR, CHSE
Assistant Professor, RNFA Subspecialty Program Coordinator, Distance Simulation Coordinator, The University of Alabama at Birmingham School of Nursing, Birmingham, Alabama, USA

Contents

Simulation is a teaching and learning strategy that is used commonly in healthcare education in academia and practice settings. Nurses at the bedside may recall times in their formal education where simulation was used as a form of clinical learning or evaluation of their performance. It is possible that with the rise of nurse residency programs and in situ simulation that bedside nurses are experiencing simulation regularly within the workplace as a means of professional development. This article will set the stage for educators to develop high-quality simulation experiences.

As healthcare providers, ethical decisions are woven into the fabric of our profession from bedside care to the use of simulation as an educational pedagogy. Simulation as a method for healthcare education began in response to ethical dilemmas in clinical practice. Educators require an interactive approach to education that will keep patients, learners, and faculty psychologically safe, decrease errors in clinical practice, and engage participants, all of which are inherent in simulation-based experiences. Professional integrity and morality are infused throughout simulation design: prebriefing, facilitation, debriefing, and evaluation.

This article provides practical recommendations for creating and implementing culturally appropriate and culturally congruent healthcare simulation applications for bedside providers that adhere to best practices and reporting standards. Framed within the 11 criteria for simulation design outlined in the Healthcare Simulation Standards of Best Practice, the article provides a summary of these criteria, highlighting the lessons learned from their application in a Health Resources and Services Administration–sponsored public health grant 6 U4EHP46217-01-01, Public Health Simulation-Infused Program.

Donna S. McDermott, Samantha Smeltzer, and Jessica L. Kamerer

Simulation is an effective method for learning and demonstrating competency in the clinical setting. Like protocols used by nurses in the practice setting, simulation educators have standards of best practice to guide their use of simulation for teaching and learning. By using the Healthcare Simulation Standard of Best Practice: Prebriefing, the simulation educators and nurse preceptors can create safe learning and working environments. Incorporating a standard prebriefing method and plan that carries throughout the clinical environment may be one way to decrease stress and anxiety of the nursing team and promote a psychologically safe working environment.

Mary K. Fey and Kate J. Morse

Debriefing is a specific type of reflective learning. Debriefing follows an experience, with the goal of taking meaningful learning away from the experience. It is often used following a simulation-based educational experience but the same techniques can be used following actual clinical care. Early studies in simulation suggest that learning does not occur in simulation-based education in the absence of debriefing. There are phases of a debriefing discussion and specific conversational strategies that are used to engage learners and provoke engaging learning discussions. Standards of practice call for facilitators with specialized training and a debriefing method that is theory based.

Darla Gruben and Elizabeth Wells-Beede

Implementing simple and effective nursing simulation experiences at the bedside or in a simulation center in a hospital setting can be an impactful way to enhance skill development, encourage critical thinking, and improve patient safety. However, there are often challenges and barriers to the bedside nurses participating in simulation in the hospital setting. Applying the Healthcare Simulation Standards of Best Practice will give the bedside nurse and educator consistency in implementing and planning effective simulations.

Carrie Westmoreland Miller, Yuting Lin, and Mary Schafer

Simulation-based education is a widely used teaching technique in healthcare education. Simulation can provide a rich learning environment for caregivers at all levels. Creating simulation-based scenarios is a systematic, evidence-based, learner-centered process that requires skill and expertise. There are 11 known criteria of best practice in simulation design. Using best practices in simulation scenario design development can provide the bedrock for learners to engage in clinical practice with competency, confidence, and caring. Examples and suggestions are provided to guide readers to create quality, learner-centered simulation scenarios using the Healthcare Simulation Standards of Best Practice: Simulation Design.

For maximum effectiveness of a simulation-based educational experience, the correct modality must be chosen. Modality refers to the equipment or platform used to conduct the simulation. There are a variety of options available to clinical simulation educators, ranging from simple task trainers to full-body manikins to virtual experiences. The correctly chosen modality will allow the learners to achieve the learning objectives.

Ineffective communication is implicated in 80% of medical errors, costing the United States approximately $12 billion annually. Teaching communication skills is a component of nursing curricula linked to improved patient outcomes. Simulation-based experience (SBE) is a strategy for healthcare professionals to learn communication skills. Providing nurses with the ability to practice nurse–nurse, nurse–physician, nurse–patient, and team communication skills in a psychologically safe learning environment provides an opportunity for skill development and meaningful self-reflection. The multiple modalities for SBE support needed communication techniques for skill development and acquisition to improve patient outcomes.

Simulation-enhanced interprofessional education (SIM-IPE) offers an avenue to teach and facilitate communication, collaboration, and teamwork while gaining an appreciation for the unique roles different healthcare professionals from a variety of settings bring to such learning experiences. This article provides an initial overview of the current trajectory of interprofessional simulation-based education in healthcare practice. An introduction to the Interprofessional Education Collaborative Core Competencies and the Healthcare Simulation Standards of Best Practice will have a TM after Practice in superscript. Practical applications of integrating Sim-IPE into the varied workplaces where nurses are leaders within interdisciplinary teams are provided.

Healthcare systems have been challenged to reduce errors, improve patient outcomes, and enhance the quality of care provided. Simulation can support patient safety and risk management by improving medical and nursing education, knowledge, skills, and behavior. This engaging experiential teaching method helps healthcare professionals identify and correct potential sources of error in their practice and has also improved safety and clinical outcomes.

Across the healthcare continuum simulation is routinely integrated into the curriculum for nurses and other professionals. The amount of simulation experienced at different points in the clinical setting highly depends on the specialty and organizational investment. The use of simulation in nursing can be divided into five specific use cases. Required and specialty certification courses include the following: Nurse Onboarding, Nurse Continuing Education, Regulatory & Joint Commission, and Interprofessional Education. Although common elements exist for each of the above-mentioned use cases, there are distinct advantages, disadvantages, and implementation challenges with each that need to be considered.

Nursing education at the undergraduate and graduate levels is undergoing a transformational curricular change that includes moving toward a competency-based curriculum. This opportunity holds promise to close the education–practice gap that has plagued nursing education for decades. A key teaching modality to achieve this outcome is simulation-based education. This article will explore the interaction between simulation and competency-based education.

The effectiveness of simulation to reduce the theory-practice gap in graduate nursing education is supported by an extensive body of research, and numerous studies have demonstrated improved learner outcomes in such areas as clinical competence, confidence, and preparedness for practice. This paper explores the types of simulation-based education available for graduate nursing programs and provides examples of graduate nursing simulations that educators can use in their own programs to prepare clinicians for practice.

NURSING CLINICS

FORTHCOMING ISSUES

December 2024
Addressing Contemporary Issues in Women's Health
Jacquelyn McMillian-Bohler and Stephanie Devane-Johnson, *Editors*

March 2025
Advances in Wound Care and Wound Management
Melania Howell, Tuba Şengül, Holly Kirkland-Kyhn, *Editors*

June 2025
Contemporary Issues in Infectious Disease: Implications for Practice
Jeffrey Kwong, *Editor*

RECENT ISSUES

June 2024
Care of People Living with HIV: Contemporary Issues
Kara S. McGee, *Editor*

March 2024
The Culture of Care
Kellie Bryant and Tiffani Chidume, *Editors*

December 2023
Trends in Men's Health
Brent MacWilliams, *Editor*

SERIES OF RELATED INTEREST

Advances in Family Practice Nursing
www.advancesinfamilypracticenursing.com

THE CLINICS ARE AVAILABLE ONLINE!
Access your subscription at:
www.theclinics.com

Foreword

Revolutionizing Simulation in Nursing Education and Practice

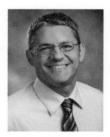

Benjamin Smallheer, PhD, RN, ACNP-BC, FNP-BC, CCRN, CNE, FAANP
Consulting Editor

Simulation, once confined to the realm of aviation and military training, has become highly integrated into nursing education, offering a dynamic platform for experiential learning. The diverse landscape of simulation modalities, from high-fidelity manne-quins to virtual-reality environments, offers a unique set of advantages in preparing nurses for the complexities of real-world practice. The term "simulation" is defined as Imitation of a situation or process, the action of pretending. From this perspective, it is hard to imagine a time when the nursing profession hasn't included some degree of simulation within its curriculum.

In the ever-evolving landscape of health care, nurses stand at the forefront, embodying the essence of compassion, skill, and innovation. The demands on nursing professionals, expanding scope of practice, and the expectation for graduates to be practice ready at graduation have grown exponentially. Therefore, so must their methods of education and training. This issue, focusing on simulation in nursing practice captures the current path toward a future where simulation technology continues to revolutionize nursing education and practice.

But "Blazing Forward" goes beyond mere description; it delves into the very essence of simulation-based education, dissecting its role in fostering critical thinking, decision-making skills, and interdisciplinary collaboration. We discuss the importance of debrief-ing, the value of simulation in clinical practice, quality and safety, and evidence-based scenario development.

As the health care landscape continues to evolve, so too must our methods of education and training. This forward-thinking issue, meticulously curated by experts in the field, serves as a testament to the transformative power of simulation across nursing education. It delves into the heart of this innovative approach, exploring its profound impact on the preparation, competency, and confidence of nursing students

Nurs Clin N Am 59 (2024) xiii–xiv
https://doi.org/10.1016/j.cnur.2024.04.001
0029-6465/24/ **nursing.theclinics.com**

and the seasoned professional. It is a call to action, urging educators, administrators, and policymakers to embrace innovation and harness the full potential of simulation in preparing the next generation of nursing leaders.

Benjamin Smallheer, PhD, RN, ACNP-BC, FNP-BC, CCRN, CNE, FAANP
Duke University School of Nursing
307 Trent Drive
DUMC Box 3322
Durham, NC 27710, USA

E-mail address:
benjamin.smallheer@duke.edu

Preface

Blazing Forward: Simulation in Nursing Practice

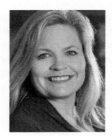

Penni I. Watts, PhD, CHSE-A, RN, FNAP, ANEF, FSSH, FAAN
Editor

The future of simulation-based education in nursing is now. Simulation is an irrefutable and imperative approach to teaching and developing nurses from academia to clinical practice, and we must embrace effective integration of its use. Simulation provides standardization of cases and promotes critical thinking without exposing patients to risks. The landscape for nurses has evolved, becoming more complex while concurrently preparing the new generation for bedside responsibilities. The utilization of simulation has emerged as a noteworthy strategy, making its presence felt in both clinical and academic settings. This becomes particularly evident in the face of challenges related to clinical placement, the identification of preceptors, and the retention of nurses at the bedside.

This issue of *Nursing Clinics of North America* is dedicated to examining simulation across the spectrum, spanning from the classroom to the clinical environment. The articles within this issue provide guidance on developing simulations while offering exemplars across diverse settings. However, many educators are implementing simulation without using best practice standards or any training. We can no longer "throw a manikin in a room and run a simulation." These articles provide evidence and align with the International Nursing Association for Clinical Simulation and Learning Healthcare Simulation Standards of Best Practice™ and program accreditation standards set by the Society for Simulation in Healthcare. As you will also see, threaded throughout this issue, professionalism in simulation is essential for all those facilitating these experiences. The Healthcare Simulationist Code of Ethics asserts key aspirational values important to the practice of simulation: Integrity, Transparency, Mutual Respect, Professionalism, Accountability, and Results Orientation.

We anticipate that this issue will offer simple yet effective strategies for best practice across all simulation implementations. Contrary to common belief, not every simulation

Nurs Clin N Am 59 (2024) xv–xvi
https://doi.org/10.1016/j.cnur.2024.02.008
0029-6465/24/© 2024 Published by Elsevier Inc.

nursing.theclinics.com

necessitates advanced technology or a high-fidelity manikin; it can transpire in a conference room or a medical-surgical ward in the hospital. Throughout this issue, the integral role of simulation in nursing education and clinical practice is apparent, including examples and case studies to support your understanding of the issue concepts. Specific examples address cultural considerations, professional development, debriefing across the curriculum and clinical settings, and the use of simulation to address quality and patient safety.

This issue of *Nursing Clinics of North America* is intended to inform simulation best practice across academia and clinical practice, engaging and educating healthcare professionals in a safe environment and preparing them to provide excellent patient care. We trust that this edition will contribute to fortifying the implementation of effective, evidence-based experiences. While this issue cannot cover every aspect of the simulation arena, we challenge you to explore additional evidence, manuscripts, and textbooks in your pursuit of developing simulations. We invite you to consider the potential of simulation and its impact.

DISCLOSURES

P.I. Watts has no disclosures or conflicts of interest.

Penni I. Watts, PhD, CHSE-A, RN, FNAP, ANEF, FSSH, FAAN
Acute, Chronic & Continuing Care
The University of Alabama at Birmingham
School of Nursing
Birmingham, AL 35294, USA

E-mail address:
piwatts@uab.edu

Creating an Effective Simulation Environment

Beth Fentress Hallmark, PhD, RN, MSN, CHSE-A, ANEF[a,*],
Brandon Kyle Johnson, PhD, RN, CHSE, ANEF[b]

KEYWORDS

- In situ • Psychological safety • Healthcare Simulation Standards of Best Practice
- Bedside simulation • Patient safety • Simulation theory

KEY POINTS

- Developing simulations should include evidence-based standards such as the Healthcare Simulation Standards of Best Practice[TM] and the Association of Standardized Patient Educators (ASPE) standards.
- There are many resources that provide guidance for simulation implementation and development, such as Society for Simulation in Healthcare (SSIH), the International Nursing Association for Clinical Simulation and Learning, and ASPE.
- Simulation leads to better patient outcomes in contrast to the lengthy waiting period between recertification.
- Evidence demonstrates that when psychological safety is *low* in-patient care settings, even when healthcare professionals are dedicated to patient safety, there are *more* errors.
- Constructivism and experiential learning theory are 2 of the primary theoretic frameworks, among many, that support simulation as a teaching and learning strategy.

INTRODUCTION

Simulation is a teaching and learning strategy that is used commonly in healthcare education in academia and practice settings. Nurses at the bedside may recall times in their formal education where simulation was used as a form of clinical learning and/or evaluation of their performance. It is possible that with the rise of nurse residency programs and in situ simulation (ISS) in the working environment that bedside nurses are experiencing simulation regularly within the workplace as a means of professional development. While there are high-cost simulators and technology, simulation conferences now boast low-cost options that yield high impact on patient outcomes. In fact, simulation is being used for a wide variety of skill attainment and decision-making

[a] Inman College of Nursing, Belmont Simulation Center, Belmont University, 1900 Belmont Boulevard, Nashville, TN 37212, USA; [b] TTUHSC Simulation Program, TTUHSC School of Nursing, Texas Tech University Health Sciences Center, 3601 4th Street, Lubbock, TX 79430, USA
* Corresponding author.
E-mail address: beth.hallmark@belmont.edu

Nurs Clin N Am 59 (2024) 345–358
https://doi.org/10.1016/j.cnur.2024.02.003   nursing.theclinics.com
0029-6465/24/© 2024 Elsevier Inc. All rights reserved.

situations. Ten years ago, the National Council of State Boards of Nursing National Simulation Study demonstrated that up to 50% of clinical time in prelicensure nursing programs could be replaced with simulation.[1] Healthcare professionals in multiple disciplines now lead teams using simulation to inform how they communicate with other members of the healthcare team.[2] Nurse simulationists demonstrated evidence that was foundational to the development of the Resuscitation Quality Improvement initiative by the American Heart Association. The researchers demonstrated, through simulation, that more frequent practice led to better patient outcomes in contrast to the lengthy waiting period between recertification.[3,4] Simulation continues to be the educational approach that is disrupting nursing, education, and healthcare, and demonstrating better outcomes.[5]

The beginnings of simulation coincided with a rapid increase in the types of technology being utilized for the simulated experiences. But simulation was never solely about the technology. In 2004, simulation pioneer David Gaba stated "Simulation is a technique-not a technology-to replace or amplify real experiences with guided experiences that evoke or replicate substantial aspects of the real world in a fully interactive manner."[6] Twenty years later, simulation is now considered a form of pedagogy,[7] contains standards of best practice,[8,9] boasts evidence-based outcomes, has avenues for accreditation and certification, and is accompanied by numerous organizations that encompass a globally and discipline-diverse membership dedicated to providing better patient care through simulation. This is because simulation is a teaching strategy that is backed with insurmountable educational theories and now a plethora of evidence supporting that it is effective for teaching clinical judgment and reasoning. Furthermore, simulation is rooted in a culture of psychological safety, or the ability to speak up without fear of retribution, which has a demonstrated impact on psychological safety.[10]

In this article, we introduce topics to create effective simulation environments that promote psychologically safe healthcare teams and contribute to safer patient outcomes. We also introduce common simulation approaches to training with simulation in practice settings. Next, a brief overview of the theoretic foundation to simulation is discussed. Finally, we provide an introduction to the Healthcare Simulation Standards of Best Practice™ (HSSOBP™) and the Association of Standardized Patient (SP) Educators (ASPE) Standards of Best Practice. Simulations that are designed with these elements in mind are foundational to high-impact and high-quality simulation-based experiences.

PATIENT SAFETY

The continuing education of nurses involves more than preparing them for the day-to-day patient care; nurses must be critical thinkers, able to interpret often obscure sets of data to provide safe and competent care to their patients while communicating effectively across many disciplines. Today's nurse must be technologically savvy and offer basic care and comfort to patients and families. Simulation provides an educational avenue for team training, identifying potential errors in systems, refining situational awareness and clinical judgment, and improving skills with the hope of improving patient outcomes.

A sentinel event is a patient safety event that results in death, permanent harm, or severe temporary harm.[11] In 2022, "failures in communications, teamwork and inconsistently following polices were the leading causes for reported sentinel events. Most reported sentinel events occurred in a hospital (88%). Of all the sentinel events, 20% were associated with patient death, 44% with severe temporary harm and 13% with unexpected additional care/extended stay".[11] Systems failures, such as overriding safety measures put in place, human factors, lack of efficiency, and staffing allocations, can lead to medical errors. Simulation can examine human and system factors. Simulations have demonstrated significance in improving performance, including being used in conducting a root cause analysis to address adverse events.[10] Collaboration between facility educators and safety committees allows for identification and remediation of errors that may lead to serious sequela for the patient and the system. Developing a simulation that recreates an error and subsequently making procedural or system changes is a first step to improving patient outcomes. Furthermore, to make an impact on patient safety, simulations that are developed according to standards of best practice are supported to build psychological safety, which has demonstrated a direct link to patient safety.[12]

In 2022, "failures in communications, teamwork and inconsistently following policies were the leading causes for reported sentinel events. Most reported sentinel events occurred in a hospital (88%). Of all the sentinel events, 20% were associated with patient death, 44% with severe temporary harm and 13% with unexpected additional care/extended stay"[13]

PSYCHOLOGICAL SAFETY

Psychological safety exists when team members are "willing and able to take the inherent interpersonal risks of candor [and] fear holding back their full participation *more* than they fear sharing a potentially sensitive, threatening, or wrong idea."[12] Nurses are often encouraged by their facilities to "speak up" about safety concerns; there is often discomfort in speaking up and a benefit to oneself to remain silent due to fear of damaging work relationships, especially when hierarchy and power perceptions among different professionals exist. Evidence demonstrates that when psychological safety is *low* in patient care settings, even when healthcare professionals are dedicated to patient safety, there are *more* errors.[12]

Psychological safety is not a new concept to simulation literature and is often referred to as a setting a safe container for learning.[14–17] Often, there is confusion about this term due to the rise of "safe spaces" which are places that are free of bias, conflict, or ideas. In a stark contrast, psychological safety is where conflicting views and ideas may be present, but the environment welcomes those thoughts and they would be met with curiosity and good feedback. In healthcare simulation, facilitators have the opportunity to design clinical situations that push learners to the edge of what they know,[18] but also model psychological safety in how the simulation is prebriefed, facilitated, and debriefed. In an environment where learners are at risk of being deceived by the clinical situation and judged by their peers,[19] high-quality simulations will hold learners both to high expectations and high regard, and facilitators model how psychologically safe teams give, receive, and come to expect good feedback.[15,20] Simulations that facilitate this kind of environment with healthy team dynamics and communication can contribute to how patient care situations are handled when conflict arises, thereby modeling behaviors that are essential to safer patient care in practice settings.

WHY SIMULATION IN THE PRACTICE ARENA?

The use of simulation as a strategy to train students in academic settings has been embraced by educators across health science disciplines has become more prevalent over the last 10 to 15 years. The evidence demonstrates that clinical performance and safety are positively impacted when simulation is used to train nurses in such skills as intravenous insertions, medication administration, neurologic examinations, hand hygiene performance, and decreases the time when asking for help.[21] While the majority of simulation-based experiences (SBEs) occurs in academic settings and many practicing nursing students experienced simulation nursing school, clinical facilities also have begun to use simulation as a tool for educating healthcare teams. Further, despite standards of best practice and due to varying state regulations, the quality and quantity of simulation a student experiences varies. In addition, most nursing students were not exposed to interprofessional simulation. Once nurses enter the workforce, the opportunity to learn and improve does not cease (**Table 1**).

Simulation at the bedside is often referred to as "in-situ" simulation. In situ is defined by the Healthcare Simulation Dictionary as "in the original place or position."[27] This is in contrast to SBEs that occur in a simulation suite or centers such as a college of nursing. ISS has many advantages including participants' familiarity with the clinical space and equipment, including the day-to-day workflow and personnel.[28] ISSs occur in clinical environments and are used to "improve knowledge, competency, and communication among providers, leading to improved patient care."[29] ISS provides the opportunity for interprofessional simulation training to occur as participation improves related to the fact that the event occurs within the clinical or work environment.[30] Disciplines that work together each day may not have had the opportunity to train together. ISS provides learners the opportunity to examine and improve communication practices, consider teamwork dynamics, investigate process design, and reflect on organizational improvements. Current evidence notes that the design, implementation, and evaluation of ISS varies. In addition, training of facilitators was not consistent with current simulation education standards, and silos and power differentials were among the concerns found in the literature.[31,32] Some basic principles of simulation pedagogy were not followed including feedback, planned debriefing practices, active learning principles, defined learning objectives, and program evaluation and ensuring an environment of psychological safety.[32] "ISS has benefits that include higher levels of contextual and environmental fidelity and convenience of access"[33] while also having inherent risks for the learner and the patients on

Table 1 Simulation in the practice arena	
In Situ Simulation	The SBE conducted in the actual patient care area/setting in which the healthcare providers would normally function to achieve a high level of fidelity.[22]
Just-In Time Training	A method of training that is conducted directly prior to a potential intervention The training that is utilized is "just-in time" at the "place near the site of the potential intervention."[23]
Nurse Residency Simulation	"Orientation through skill-based learning, critical thinking, human factors engineering, and patient safety using simulated experiences for a wide variety of high-risk, low-frequency, as well as high-frequency, commonly occurring clinical events and situations."[24]
Team-based Training	Simulation that is used to "successfully transfer the knowledge skills and attiitudes (KSAs) to the clinical arena and to improve patient safety."[25]
Resuscitation Training	Uses rapid cycle deliberate practice, mastery learning, and scripted feedback to improve resuscitation.[26]

the unit.[34] The pressures that are unavoidable within patient care areas such as the need for a bed for a patient, patient acuity, and staffing needs all may be seen as barriers to ISS. While there may be risk involved, understanding how to create an effective simulation environment can help mitigate that risk and provide a powerful tool for learners.

Another application of ISS is "just-in time" training where nurses are retrained on a skill immediately prior to performing the skill. "Simulation is widely accepted in hospital orientation and transition-to-practice programs because it has been shown to increase knowledge, improve communication, and provide educators with the ability to measure clinical judgment in real-time."[35] There has been a long history of using simulation for resuscitation training in the acute care environment. The advanced cardiovascular life support, basic life support, pediatric advanced life support, and Neonatal Resuscitation Program have used SBE since their inception. For many types of simulation-based training, a step that may be ignored is the feedback and time for reflection facilitated by a trained educator. Understanding the theoretic foundations, HSSOBP™, ASPE standards, accreditation criteria, and certification opportunities is the key to implementing a successful simulation program.

THEORETIC SUPPORT

Constructivism and experiential learning theory are two of the primary theoretic frameworks, among many, which support simulation as a teaching and learning strategy. Constructivism, based on Piaget's research in child development, is based strongly on the foundation that learners construct new ideas, building on their previous experiences and knowledge.[36] The goals of a practice profession such as nursing include assimilation (how knowledge fits with previously developed schema) and accommodation (how knowledge develops when opposing to existing frames).[36,37]

Assimilation and accommodation are 2 foundational outcomes of experiential learning. Experiential learning is defined by Kolb as "the process whereby knowledge is created through the transformation of experience. Knowledge results from the combination of grasping and transforming experience."[38] It has been demonstrated that learners who are both in participatory hands-on roles, and those in observational roles, experience the cyclical nature of experiential learning and have similar learning outcomes.[39,40] A learner grasps, or takes in the experience, through participating in an SBE clinical care, and debriefing methods help learners transform the experience by providing a space for learners to reflect, consider new strategies through abstract conceptualization and finally there is application of the new knowledge/strategies during the active experimentation phase. This entire cycle is the transformational experience that Kolb defined (**Table 2**).

The following section addresses the HSSOBP™ and the ASPE Standards of Practice. Simulation facilitators can be certain that when following these standards of practice, they are building simulations that are founded strongly on educational theory.

STANDARDS OF BEST PRACTICE
Healthcare Simulation Standards of Best Practice

The HSSOBP™ are living documents that are updated regularly citing evidence from published research.[8] Nurses and other healthcare professionals are being onboarded using simulation to demonstrate competence. There is an expectation that simulation will be a part of the transition to practice. In addition, the staff of healthcare facilities may be exposed to simulation as part of their ongoing professional development.[33] The evolution of simulation as a tool in the education of healthcare professionals

Table 2 Assimilation and accommodation	
Assimilation	A nurse receives a handoff report to care for a patient with congestive heart failure. The nurse hears bilateral crackles in lung fields and determines there is pitting edema. This finding is similar to what the nurse read about congestive heart failure in textbooks and learned about in classroom environments.
Accommodation	A nurse administers pain medication to a patient complaining of 4/10 pain that is aching and throbbing postoperatively. After 30 min, the patient is now complaining of pain that is 7/10 that is now sharp and radiating. The nurse decides to notify the provider rather than attempting another pain medication, as the nurse is anticipating the cause of pain may be something different.

has been documented in the evidence and is growing rapidly.[11] Simulation is just that a tool. Tools, when used correctly, can make the job much easier and more efficient. Tools can also harm and cause trauma when standards are not followed and instructions not heeded. Standards provide the user with guidelines for effective use and give the user a benchmark to follow. Since 2011, the HSSOBP™ have been providing simulationists with this type of benchmark. The standards, previously known as the International Nursing Association for Clinical Simulation and Learning standards, have been revised and updated over the past 12 years based on new evidence and pedagogical guidelines. **Table 3** provides a list of each of the HSSOBP™.

These standards of best practice were developed by interprofessional teams of simulationists and guide both academicians and clinicians in the design, implementation, and evaluation of simulation experiences. When designing simulation for the bedside professional, it is essential to consider the HSSOBP™. Essential components of these standards are a foundation to working toward high-quality simulations and experiences that foster psychological safety. Simulation in an academic setting may integrate these standards differently than they would be used for simulation in a practice setting; however, it is imperative that they are considered in all environments (**Box 1**).

Association of Standardized Patient Educators Standards of Best Practice

A SP is an individual who is trained to take on the character of a patient or family member. "In more recent years, SPs may portray an expanded scope of roles (eg, clients, family members, healthcare professionals). There is increasing recognition that SP methodology can be applied to the work of any individual portraying a human in any simulation modality (eg, confederates, learners playing roles other than themselves, technicians operating a manikin)."[9] SPs are mostly employed in academic settings; however, SPs have been utilized in simulation-based events that examine safety threats, communication among team members, and system issues.[50] Nursing educators in practice settings may be asked to develop these types of events, while ensuring the safety of participants, the SPs, and the patients and their families is critical. The ASPE has published a set of standards for simulationist to follow during the design and implementation of simulation events.[9] **Table 4** provides a list of the ASPE standards which are divided by domains and supported by principles to follow.

The HSSOBP™ and ASPE Standards of Practice are 2 sets of standards that are essential to developing simulations with high impact and an effective simulation

Table 3
The Healthcare Simulation Standards of Best Practice

Standard	Application to Bedside Simulation
Professional Development[22]	• Align professional goals with organizational goals. • Provide evidence for return on investment related to conferences and other continued education (CE) events. • Partner with system-wide individuals in finance, education, risk management, and accreditation to advocate for simulation professional development and funding.
Prebriefing[41]	• Provide orientation to physical environment including manikins and equipment functionality, even during ISS when setting is familiar. • Design a psychologically safe environment by including statements about realism, confidentiality, mutual respect, trust, and addressing hierarchy to encourage a leveled field for learning. • Communicate to learners that simulation is a safe place where mistakes are embraced, learning is the objective, and high-quality feedback will be modeled. Consider a script for consistency.
Simulation Design[42]	• Design simulations with a focus on the "why" while understanding the learner's level of experience. • Focus on team-based training, patient safety, communication, scenarios specific to certain units (eg, code simulations on a floor that may have had poor code outcomes), systems issues, human factors, and patient types. • Consult with unit experts and consider whose perspectives need to be heard to provide a simulation that is realistic. • Pilot test the scenario prior to full implementation.
Facilitation[43]	• Identify a facilitator that is proficient in knowledge and skills of simulation pedagogy, including prebriefing and debriefing, which will lead the simulation from design to evaluation. • Provide structure to the simulation by implementing consistent and realistic cues to help participants meet learning objectives. • Consider that bedside simulation events may include learners from varying levels of experience resulting in multiple pathways occurring to meet learning objectives.
The Debriefing Process[44]	• Select a facilitator that is trained in debriefing and/or feedback methodology. • Choose a debriefing method to adopt in your facility. Debriefing is not a time to teach, but to foster high-quality feedback and reflection. • Communicate debriefing findings that reveal system-related problems to administration or safety office (Maxworthy)
Operations[45]	• Develop a strategic plan, based on organizational goals and initiatives such as patient safety, team training, and systems issues. • Develop policy and procedure for equipment maintenance, equipment sharing across departments, video use, "no-go" ISS, and evaluation methods.

(continued on next page)

Table 3 (continued)	
Standard	**Application to Bedside Simulation**
	• Work with hospital safety committees to determine simulation design needs, technology needs, and data that should be collected.
Outcomes and Objectives[46]	• Align outcomes in practice settings with unit-specific goals that are tied to institutional goals. • Create objectives that are measurable and will demonstrate impact on patient care data, sentinel events, and other data the institution gathers. • Base the simulation modality and technology on learner objectives. Avoid purchasing high-cost technology without strong objectives and needs based on outcomes of the institution.
Professional Integrity[47]	• Adopt the Healthcare Simulation Code of Ethics to address mutual respect during interprofessional simulation experiences to avoid unintended power dynamics. • Design simulations with transparency in mind without the intention to "trick" the participants. • Stress the importance of confidentiality and psychological safety as participants may be fearful of an impact on their job if they perform poorly in simulation.
Simulation-Enhanced Interprofessional Education (IPE)[48]	• Include team members from all disciplines represented in the development of interprofessional simulations from the design phase to evaluation phase. • Examine practice guidelines from each discipline. • Develop objectives for each participant group.
Evaluation of Learning and Performance[49]	• Use formative evaluation approaches in practice settings for routine learning situations with a focus on feedback and reflective practice. • Inform participants of evaluation methods. • Consider evaluation of new hires for readiness to practice in nurse residency.

Box 1
THE HEALTHCARE SIMULATION STANDARDS OF BEST PRACTICE

Professional Development[22]

Prebriefing: Preparation and Briefing[41]

Simulation Design[42]

Facilitation[43]

The Debriefing Process[44]

Operations[45]

Outcomes and Objectives[46]

Professional Integrity[47]

Simulation-Enhanced Interprofessional Education[48]

Evaluation of Learning and Performance[49]

Table 4
Association of standardized patient educators standards of best practice

Domain	Principles	Application to Bedside Simulation
1.0 Safe Work Practices[9]	1.1 Safe work Environment 1.2 Confidentiality 1.3 Respect	• Consider safety issues specific to beside: medications, confidentiality, privacy, equipment that may be "real" • Inform patients of simulated events on the unit • Provide logistical details inherent to clinical areas that may differ from academia
2.0 Case Development[9]	2.1 Preparation 2.2 Case Components	• Avoid stereotyping in case development. Consult an expert. • Pilot the scenario. If not in situ give opportunity for questions and pilot elsewhere • Provide same props and materials as in academia
3.0 SP Training[9]	3.1 Preparation for Training 3.2 Training for role portrayal 3.3 Training for feedback 3.4 Training for completion of assessment instruments 3.5 Reflection on the training process	• Provide SP with learner objectives • Train for accuracy • Discuss SPs role in feedback • Provide time for practice and feedback on performance as needed for changes
4.0 Program Management[9]	4.1 Purpose 4.2 Expertise 4.3 Policies and Procedures 4.4 Record Management 4.5 Team Management 4.6 Quality Management	• Develop policies and procedures specific to SBE (in situ, disaster, residency) • Work with risk management related to unit-based simulations considering risks to patients, families and SP • Develop policies to ensure psychological safety of SP, patient and families • Consider diversity and inclusion during recruitment
5.0 Professional Development[9]	5.1 Career Development 5.2 Scholarship 5.3 Leadership	• Ensure educators are trained in SP methodology • Encourage membership in professional organizations • Develop a plan for professional growth and development specific to the practice arena

---

Box 2
Resources for simulationists

1. Society for Simulation in Healthcare (SSH)
   a. Certified Healthcare Simulation Educator Blueprint
   b. Accreditation Standards
   c. International Meeting on Simulation in Healthcare

2. Healthcare Simulation Standards of Best Practice™

3. International Nursing Association for Clinical Simulation and Learning (INACSL)
   a. Endorsement Criteria
   b. Cornerstone Education Program
   c. INACSL Simulation Conference

4. National League for Nursing (NLN)
   a. Simulation Innovation Resource Center (SIRC) courses
   b. NLN Summit

5. The Association for Standardized Patient Educators
   a. Standards of Best Practice
   b. ASPE Conference

6. National Organization of Nurse Practitioner Faculties (NONPF)
   a. Simulation Guidelines
   b. 2023 Guide to Developing Simulation

7. Canadian Alliance of Nurse Educators
   a. Competencies
   b. They also have a certification: the CCSNE

8. Association for Simulated Practice in Healthcare
   a. The ASPiH Standards 2023

9. Global Network for Simulation in Healthcare (GNSH)

---

environment. In addition, in **Box 2**, we provide additional resources for ongoing simulation professional development.

THE IMPLICATIONS OF SIMULATIONS WITHOUT STANDARDS FOR EFFECTIVE SIMULATION ENVIRONMENT

As previously mentioned, simulation has been embraced in nursing education. Clinical site scarcity and shortage of nursing faculty has accelerated this adoption resulting in state boards of nursing allowing for simulation to replace clinical hours in nursing programs.[51] While this work focuses on simulation at the bedside, it is important to provide some lessons learned from academia over the last 10 to 15 years so that simulation in practice-based settings avoids potential pitfalls.

There has been a loud cry for nursing faculty to provide a safe place for students to learn, both from simulationists and hospital educators. Many nursing students and faculty have voiced their concerns about "training scars" that have resulted from simulations that were facilitated by *untrained* faculty. After a somewhat viral social media post called out the abuse of nursing students in simulation, Kardong-Edgren and Wells-Beede write that without specific training in simulation and adherence to standards and guidelines "the psychological ramifications are substantial and may contribute to the current high burnout in nursing."[52] Nursing educators in facilities must be aware of this as they plan nurse residencies and future continuing education. Providing an effective simulation program for nurses in practice includes planning and developing experiences that integrate the HSSOBP™, the ASPE standards, and the SSH accreditation criteria.

SUMMARY

Simulation is a form of education and clinical training that, when designed correctly, has the track record to improve knowledge, skills, and attitudes about effective patient care. Further, when using standards of practice, simulation has demonstrated evidence of fostering psychologically safe spaces for equipping learners with tools to speak up in high-stress clinical situations. Psychologically safe arenas are well supported to impact patient safety. As bedside nurses pursue simulation training through continuous professional development, rest assured that while creating an effective simulation environment takes time and commitment, it contributes to effective patient care environment both for the healthcare professional teams and the patients they serve.

CLINICS CARE POINTS

- When using standards of practice, simulation has demonstrated evidence of fostering psychologically safe spaces for equipping learners with tools to speak up in high-stress clinical situations.
- While there are high-cost simulators and technology, simulation conferences now boast low-cost options that yield high impact on patient outcomes.
- Collaboration between facility educators and safety committees allows for identification and remediation of errors that may lead to serious sequela for the patient and the system.
- Simulation at the bedside is often referred to as "in situ" simulation.
- The HSSOBP™ were developed by interprofessional teams of simulationists and guide both academicians and clinicians in the design, implementation, and evaluation of simulation experiences.

DISCLOSURE

The authors have nothing to disclose.

REFERENCES

1. Hayden JK, Smiley RA, Alexander M, et al. The NCSBN national simulation study: A longitudinal, randomized, controlled study replacing clinical hours with simulation in prelicensure nursing education. Journal of Nursing Regulation 2014;5(2): S1–41.
2. Reed T, Horsley TL, Muccino K, et al. Simulation using TeamSTEPPS to promote interprofessional education and collaborative practice. Nurse Educat 2017; 42(3):E1–5.
3. American Heart Association, Resuscitation Quality Improvement Program, Available at: http://cpr.heart.org/AHAECC/CPRAndECC/Training/RQI/UCM_476470_ RQI.jsp. Accessed October 22, 2023.
4. Kardong-Edgren S, Oermann MH, Odom-Maryon T. Findings from a nursing student CPR study: implications for staff development educators. J Nurses Staff Dev 2012;28(1):9–15.

5. Waxman KT, Bowler F, Forneris SG, et al. Simulation as a nursing education disrupter. Nurs Adm Q 2019;43(4):300–5.
6. Gaba DM. The future vision of simulation in health care. Quality and Safety in Health Care 2004;13(suppl_1):i2–10.
7. Jeffries P.R., Rodgers B. and Adamson K., NLN Jeffries simulation theory: Brief narrative description, In: Jeffries P.R., *The NLN Jeffries simulation theory*, Wolters-Kluwer, the Netherlands, 2016, 292–293.
8. Standards Committee INACSL. Healthcare Simulation Standards of Best Practice™. Clinical Simulation in Nursing 2021;58(66). https://doi.org/10.1016/j.ecns.2021.08.018.
9. Lewis KL, Bohnert CA, Gammon WL, et al. The Association of Standardized Patient Educators (ASPE) Standards of Best Practice (SOBP). Adv Simul (Lond) 2017;2(1):10.
10. Bienstock J, Heuer A. A review on the evolution of simulation-based training to help build a safer future. Medicine (Baltim) 2022;101(25):e29503. https://doi.org/10.1097/md.0000000000029503.
11. The Joint Commission (2014). Summary of Sentinel Events. Available at: https://www.jointcommission.org/resources/sentinel-event/sentinel-event-data-summary/. Accessed October 20, 2023.
12. Edmondson A. The Fearless organization: creating psychological safety in the workplace for learning, Innovationand Growth. Hoboken, NJ: Wiley & Sons, Inc; 2019.
13. The Joint Commission (2014). Summary of Sentinel Events. Available at: https://www.jointcommission.org/resources/sentinel-event/sentinel-event-data-summary/. Accessed October 20, 2023.
14. Daniels AL, Morse C, Breman R. Psychological safety in simulation-based prelicensure nursing education: A narrative review. Nurse Educat 2021;46(5):E99–102.
15. Rudolph JW, Simon R, Dufresne RL, et al. There is no such thing as "nonjudgmental" debriefing: A theory and method for debriefing with good judgment. Simulat Healthc J Soc Med Simulat 2006;1(1):47–55.
16. Rudolph JW, Simon R, Rivard P, et al. Debriefing with good judgment: Combining rigorous feedback with genuine inquiry. Anesthesiol Clin 2007;25(2):361–76.
17. Rudolph JW, Raemer DB, Simon R. Establishing a safe container for learning in simulation: The role of the presimulation briefing. Simulat Healthc J Soc Med Simulat 2014;9(6):339–49.
18. Vygotsky L. Thought and Language. Cambridge, MA: MIT Press; 1986.
19. Brazil V, Purdy E. 'Safe, not soft'—Hitting the sweet spot for simulation-based education. ICE Blog blog; 2020.
20. Rock LK, Rudolph JW, Fey MK, et al. "Circle up": Workflow adaptation and psychological support via briefing, debriefing, and peer support. NEJM Catalyst 2020. https://doi.org/10.1056/cat.20.0240.
21. El Hussein MT, Hirst SP. High-Fidelity Simulation's Impact on Clinical Reasoning and Patient Safety: A Scoping Review. Journal of Nursing Regulation 2023;13(4):54–65.
22. Hallmark B, Brown M, Peterson DT, et al. Healthcare Simulation Standards of Best PracticeTM Professional Development. Clinical Simulation in Nursing 2021;58:5–8.
23. Maxworthy JC, Palaganas JC, Epps CA, et al. Defining Excellence in simulation programs. Philadelphia, PA: Lippincott Williams & Wilkins; 2022.

24. Beyea SC, von Reyn LK, Slattery MJ. A nurse residency program for competency development using human patient simulation. Journal for nurses in professional development 2007;23(2):77–82.
25. Stephen D., Pratt B, & Sachs B., Team training: Classroom training vs HighFidelity Simulation. Available at: https://psnet.ahrq.gov/perspective/team-training-classroom-training-vs-high-fidelity-simulation 2006. Accessed October 20, 2023.
26. Weiss KE, Kolbe M, Nef A, et al. Data-driven resuscitation training using pose estimation. Adv Simul (Lond). 2023;8(1):12.
27. Lioce L, Lopreiato J, Founding Ed, Downing D, Chang TP, Robertson JM, Anderson M, Diaz DA, Spain AE, Terminology and Concepts Working Group. Healthcare simulation Dictionary –Second Edition. Rockville, MD: Agency for Healthcare Research and Quality; 2020. p. 2020. AHRQ Publication No. 20-0019.
28. Nucci A, Sforzi I, Morley-Fletcher A, et al. Quality improvement initiative using blended in situ simulation training on procedural sedation and analgesia in a pediatric emergency department: better patient care at lower costs. Simulat Healthc J Soc Med Simulat 2022;17(5):299–307.
29. Tapia V., Waseem M., Setup and Execution of In Situ Simulation. [Updated 2023 May 1]. In: StatPearls [Internet]. Treasure Island (FL): StatPearls Publishing; 2024. Available at: https://www.ncbi.nlm.nih.gov/books/NBK551657/
30. Truchot J, Boucher V, Raymond-Dufresne É, et al. Evaluation of the feasibility and impacts of in situ simulation in emergency medicine—a mixed-method study protocol. BMJ Open 2021;11(3):e040360.
31. Bryn Baxendale KE, Cowley A, Bramley L, et al. GENESISS 1—Generating Standards for In-Situ Simulation project: a scoping review and conceptual model. BMC Med Educ 2022;22(479):1–18.
32. Ju M, Bochatay N, Robertson K, et al. From ideal to real: a qualitative study of the implementation of in situ interprofessional simulation-based education. BMC Med Educ 2022;22(1):301.
33. Morse C, Fey M, Kardong-Edgren S, et al. The Changing Landscape of Simulation-Based Education. Am J Nurs 2019;119(8):42–8.
34. Bajaj K, Minors A, Walker K, et al. "No-Go Considerations" for In Situ Simulation Safety. Simul Healthc 2018;13(3):221–4.
35. Klenke-Borgmann L, Mattson N, Peterman M, et al. The Long-Term Transferability of Clinical Judgment Via In-Class Simulations to Nursing Practice: A Qualitative Descriptive Study. Clinical Simulation in Nursing 2023;85. https://doi.org/10.1016/j.ecns.2023.101468.
36. Piaget J, Cook MT. The origins of intelligence in children. Madison, CT: International University Press; 1952.
37. Dreifuerst KT. The essentials of debriefing in simulation learning: A concept analysis. Nurs Educ Perspect 2009;30(2):109–14.
38. Kolb DA. Experiential learning: experience as the source of learning and development. 2nd ed. Upper Saddle River, NJ: Pearson Education, Inc; 2015.
39. Johnson BK. Simulation observers learn the same as participants: The evidence. Clinical Simulation in Nursing 2019;33(C):26–34.
40. Johnson BK. Observational experiential learning: Theoretical support for observer roles in health care simulation. J Nurs Educ 2020;59(1):7–14.
41. McDermott DS, Ludlow J, Horsley E, et al. Healthcare Simulation Standards of Best PracticeTM Prebriefing: Preparation and Briefing. Clinical Simulation in Nursing 2021;58:9–13.
42. Watts PI, McDermott DS, Alinier G, et al. Healthcare Simulation Standards of Best PracticeTM Simulation Design. Clinical Simulation in Nursing 2021;58:14–21.

43. Persico L, Belle A, DiGregorio H, et al. Healthcare Simulation Standards of Best PracticeTM Facilitation. Clinical Simulation in Nursing 2021;58:22–6.

44. Decker S, Alinier G, Crawford SB, et al. Healthcare Simulation Standards of Best PracticeTM The Debriefing Process. Clinical Simulation in Nursing 2021;58: 27–32.

45. Charnetski M, Jarvill M. Healthcare Simulation Standards of Best PracticeTM Operations. Clinical Simulation in Nursing 2021;58:33–9.

46. Miller C, Deckers C, Jones M, et al. Healthcare Simulation Standards of Best PracticeTM Outcomes and Objectives. Clinical Simulation in Nursing 2021;58:40–4.

47. Bowler F, Klein M, Wilford A. Healthcare Simulation Standards of Best PracticeTM Professional Integrity. Clinical Simulation in Nursing 2021;58:45–8.

48. Rossler K, Molloy MA, Pastva AM, et al. Healthcare Simulation Standards of Best PracticeTM Simulation-Enhanced Interprofessional Education. Clinical Simulation in Nursing 2021;58:49–53.

49. McMahon E, Jimenez FA, Lawrence K, et al. Healthcare Simulation Standards of Best PracticeTM Evaluation of Learning and Performance. Clinical Simulation in Nursing 2021;58:54–6.

50. Patterson MD, Geis GL, Falcone RA, et al. In situ simulation: detection of safety threats and teamwork training in a high risk emergency department. BMJ Qual Saf 2013;22(6):468–77.

51. Bradley CS, Johnson BK, Dreifuerst KT, et al. Regulation of Simulation Use in United States Prelicensure Nursing Programs. Clinical Simulation in Nursing 2019;33:17–25.

52. Stop Prelicensure Student Abuse in Simulation, Available at: https://simzine. news/focus-en/sim-nurse-en/stop-prelicensure-student-abuse-in-simulation/. Accessed November 1, 2023.

Professional Integrity and Ethical Considerations in Simulation

Fara Bowler, DNP, APRN, CHSE*, Patrick Luna, MSN, RN, CEN,
Tammy Spencer, DNP, RN, CNE, ACNS-BC, CCNS

KEYWORDS

- Healthcare ethics • Simulation ethics • Psychological safety • Facilitator
- Professional integrity

KEY POINTS

- Healthcare Simulationist Code of Ethics defines professional practice for simulationists.
- Psychological safety is an ethical responsibility in simulation.
- Professional integrity encompasses the Healthcare Simulationist Code of Ethics; discipline-specific code of ethics; diversity, equity, and inclusion; psychological safety; and confidentiality.

INTRODUCTION

As healthcare providers, ethical decisions are woven into the fabric of our profession from bedside care to the use of simulation as an educational pedagogy. Simulation as a method for healthcare education began in response to ethical dilemmas in clinical practice.[1] Educators require an interactive approach to education that will keep patients, learners, and faculty psychologically safe, decrease errors in clinical practice, and engage participants, all of which are inherent in simulation-based experiences (SBEs). Professional integrity and morality are infused throughout simulation design: prebriefing, facilitation, debriefing, and evaluation. Ethical knowledge, skills, and attitudes should also be applied from start to finish of an SBE with the goal of a safer, more competent healthcare delivery.

There are several seminal resources that establish ethical frameworks used in the design of a simulation program. These frameworks help to establish a professional identity within the specialty area of simulation. This article covers the impact and shared knowledge from the Healthcare Simulationist Code of Ethics[2]; Healthcare Simulation Standards of Best Practice™ (HSSOBP)™: Professional Integrity[3]; and

College of Nursing, University of Colorado, 13120 East 19th Avenue, Aurora, CO 80045, USA
* Corresponding author.
E-mail address: Fara.bowler@cuanschutz.edu

Nurs Clin N Am 59 (2024) 359–370
https://doi.org/10.1016/j.cnur.2024.02.011
0029-6465/24/© 2024 Elsevier Inc. All rights reserved.

nursing.theclinics.com

the Association of Standardized Patient Educators (ASPE) Standards of Best Practice (SOBP).[4] Ethical considerations when implementing simulation in clinical and educational settings utilize these core values inherent in the practice of simulation. By providing a meaningful SBE, educators can bring the tenants of moral reasoning to the forefront of the learner. Subsequently, these concepts will authentically be present in the learner's consciousness while they navigate the ever-changing complexities in the in clinical practice.

The Healthcare Simulationist Code of Ethics was created in 2018 by an international healthcare simulation professional workgroup convened by the Society of Simulation in Healthcare.[2] These values are essential for the welfare of all parties and applicable to everyone involved in an SBE, including but not limited to the facilitator, learner, simulated participant, and operations specialist. The aspirational values included in the Code of Ethics are integrity, transparency, mutual respect, professionalism, accountability, and results orientation and are further defined in **Table 1**.

The International Nursing Association for Clinical Simulation and Learning leads the authorship of the HSSOBP™. Professional integrity is defined in the HSSOBP™ as "ethical behaviors that are expected in simulation experiences by all parties involved."[3] In the 2021 publication of the HSSOBP™: Professional Integrity, the Healthcare Simulationist Code of Ethics was adopted and integrated into the HSSOBP™. This is a noteworthy alignment and acknowledgment of the importance of establishing the ethical framework within simulation.

There is an explicit expectation of inclusivity in the HSSOBP™: Professional Integrity. It guides staff, faculty, and learners to respect equity, diversity, and inclusivity among all involved and in all aspects of the SBE. While this may be assumed when discussing ethics in simulation, HSSOBP™: Professional Integrity was intentionally added as an independent criterion to stress the importance of this imperative in all SBEs. Being honest, mindful, and sensitive to all differences and ethical issues related to the simulation experience is necessary to create the meaningful experiences that educators strive to offer learners.[3] Holding diverse worldviews and individual differences that characterize patients, populations, and the healthcare team is a foundational viewpoint in creating an inclusive SBE.[3] See **Fig. 1** for all of the criterion included in the HSSOBP™: Professional Integrity.

Table 1 Healthcare simulationist code of ethics	
Integrity	Maintain the highest standards of integrity including honesty, truthfulness, fairness, and judgment.
Transparency	Perform simulation activities in a manner that promotes transparency and clarity in the design, communication, and decision-making processes.
Mutual Respect	Respect the rights, dignity, and worth of all and practice empathy and compassion to support beneficence and nonmaleficence toward all involved in simulation activities.
Professionalism	Demonstrate professional competence, engage in professional development, and develop new entrants to the profession.
Accountability	Be accountable for decisions and actions while role modeling ethical behavior.
Results Orientation	Support simulation activities that enhance the quality of the healthcare profession. Activities should be directed toward achievable outcomes that directly impact healthcare practice and systems.

From Society for Simulation in Healthcare (2018) Healthcare Simulationist Code of Ethics. Available at http://www.ssih.org/Code-of-Ethics. Used with permission.

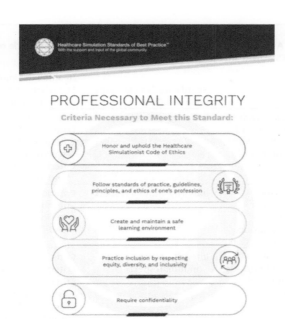

Fig. 1. Healthcare simulation standards of best practice™: PROFESSIONAL integrity. (*From* INACSL Standards Committee, Bowler, F., Klein, M. & Wilford, A. Healthcare Simulation Standards of Best Practice™ Professional Integrity. Clin Sim 2021; 58, 45-48. https://doi. org/10.1016/j.ecns.2021.08.014. Used with permission.)

The values presented in the Healthcare Simulationist Code of Ethics and the HSSOBP™: Professional Integrity intersect with the American Nurses Association (ANA) Code of Ethics[5] and provide a template for ethical practice in nursing simulation. In **Table 2**, the Healthcare Simulationist Code of Ethics and the HSSOBP™: Professional Integrity are mapped to the ANA Code of Ethics to demonstrate the relationships between these fundamental ethical expectations. The 9 provisions in the ANA Code of Ethics can map to the Healthcare Simulationist Code of Ethics and HSSOBP™ to illustrate how the overall practice of healthcare simulation can be implemented using values inherent to nursing practice.

The results of this ethical crosswalk yield a theme of integrity and mutual respect as being the most frequently aligned Healthcare Simulationist Code of Ethics values with the ANA Code of Ethics. This alignment reflects the patient-centered focus of nursing care and highlights how nursing simulation can be implemented to reflect the ethical values of the profession. It also illustrates the nursing profession's dedication to diversity, inclusion, and an awareness of healthcare provider bias.

Sound ethical decision-making can be cultivated in simulation environments and directly influence clinical practice.[6] Patient-centered SBEs that allow learners to display nursing values such as advocacy, empathy, and nursing autonomy can prepare nurses for ethical decision-making in practice. This education can also be expanded to include experiences that highlight how to effectively communicate within interprofessional teams regarding ethical decisions and safe patient care.[6]

The facilitator of a simulation experience faces an initial ethical challenge with the decision to adopt simulation as a modality to improve nursing practice. Given the mounting literature on the efficacy of simulation, the question becomes: is it a violation

Table 2
American Nurses Association Code of Ethics,[5] Healthcare Simulationist Code of Ethics,[2] and HSSOBP™: PROFESSIONAL integrity[3] crosswalk

ANA Code of Ethics	Healthcare Simulationist Code of Ethics	Healthcare Simulation Standards of Best Practice™: Professional Integrity
1. The nurse practices with compassion and respect for the inherent dignity, worth, and unique attributes of every person	Integrity, mutual respect	Criterion 1: Code of ethics Criterion 2: Ethics of profession Criterion 3: Safe learning environment Criterion 4: Diversity, equity, and inclusion
2. The nurse's primary commitment is to the patient, whether an individual, family, group, community, or population.	Integrity, mutual respect	Criterion 1: Code of ethics Criterion 2: Ethics of profession Criterion 4: Diversity, equity, and inclusion
3. The nurse promotes, advocates for, and protects the rights, health, and safety of the patient.	Integrity, transparency, mutual respect	Criterion 1: Code of ethics Criterion 2: Ethics of profession Criterion 3: Safe learning environment Criterion 4: Diversity, equity, and inclusion
4. The nurse has authority, accountability, and responsibility for nursing practice; makes decisions; and takes action consistent with the obligation to provide optimal patient care.	Integrity, professionalism, accountability	Criterion 1: Code of ethics Criterion 2: Ethics of profession
5. The nurse owes the same duties to self as to others, including the responsibility to promote health and safety, preserve wholeness of character and integrity, maintain competence, and continue personal and professional growth.	Mutual respect, professionalism, accountability	Criterion 1: Code of ethics Criterion 2: Ethics of profession
6. The nurse, through individual and collective effort, establishes, maintains, and improves the ethical environment of the work setting and conditions of employment that are conducive to safe, quality healthcare.	Integrity, transparency, results orientation	Criterion 1: Code of ethics Criterion 2: Ethics of profession Criterion 3: Safe learning environment Criterion 4: Diversity, equity, and inclusion

(*continued on next page*)

		Healthcare Simulation
	Healthcare Simulationist	Standards of Best Practice™:
ANA Code of Ethics	Code of Ethics	Professional Integrity
7. The nurse, in all roles and settings, advances the profession through research and scholarly inquiry, professional standards development, and the generation of both nursing and health policy.	Professionalism, accountability, results orientation	Criterion 1: Code of ethics Criterion 2: Ethics of profession
8. The nurse collaborates with other health professionals and the public to protect human rights, promote health diplomacy, and reduce health disparities.	Integrity, mutual respect	Criterion 1: Code of ethics Criterion 2: Ethics of profession Criterion 3: Safe learning environment Criterion 4: Diversity, equity, and inclusion Criterion 5: Academic integrity
9. The profession of nursing, collectively through its professional organizations, must articulate nursing values, maintain the integrity of the profession, and integrate principles of social justice into nursing and health policy.	Integrity, mutual respect	Criterion 1: Code of ethics Criterion 2: Ethics of profession Criterion 4: Diversity, equity, and inclusion

Table 2
(continued)

Data from American Nurses Association. Code of ethics for nurses with interpretive statements. Nursesbooks.org [5]; 2015, Society for Simulation in Healthcare (2018) Healthcare Simulationist Code of Ethics,[2] HSSOBP™: Professional Integrity (2021).[3]

of ethical principles to avoid adoption of simulation experiences to improve nursing practice? The ANA Code of Ethics[5] focuses on competence in practice and accountability for decision-making. Simulation experiences have proven efficacy in both these areas.[6] Therefore, is it ethical and equitable for some learners to have access to simulation experiences while others do not?

The simulation facilitator is subsequently charged with creating an environment conducive to learning and utilizing ethical standards. Simulation experiences can be inherently anxiety and stress producing. These emotions can have a negative impact on the learner's behavior and outcomes.[7] A critical component of creating a safe learning environment is fostering psychological safety. Psychological safety is defined as learners feeling comfortable participating, speaking up, sharing thoughts, and asking for help as needed without concern for retribution or embarrassment.[7] This definition can be linked to the ANA Code of Ethics Provision 5, which focuses on nurses respecting themselves and each other with the same ethical principles that they would apply to a patient.[5] Psychological safety can also be attributed to the original ethical question that resulted in the methodology of simulation being adopted in healthcare. Fostering psychologically safe environments achieves the original aim of keeping all participants safe. Conversely, not creating a psychologically safe environment will negatively impact student engagement and outcomes that may be directly related to patient safety.[7]

ASPE addresses ethical responsibilities specific to standardized patients in the ASPE SOBP Domain 1: Safe work environment. There are 3 distinct principles related to creating a safe work environment: safe work practices, confidentiality, and respect.[4] The concept of mutual respect is threaded throughout the literature as an ethical construct integral to simulation.

According to the NLN Jeffries Simulation Theory, there is a dynamic interaction between the simulation facilitator and participant that occurs within an SBE.[8] For this relationship to achieve the intended simulation outcomes, the SBE must occur in an environment with established trust. The responsibility for creating this trust lies with both facilitator and participant. Utilizing this framework, the facilitator should understand that the creation of the psychologically safe environment is not solely the responsibility of the facilitator and is a collaborative effort with the learners.[8] This becomes vitally important when it is understood that it is the learners' perspective of psychological safety that ultimately determines whether this environment has been created.[7] For example, a facilitator may believe that they have created a psychologically safe environment for a simulation, but still may not achieve simulation outcomes due to lack of safety or trust experienced by learners. Psychological safety is a uniquely lived experience of the facilitator and learner.

Learner perspectives of what fosters psychological safety and positive learner outcomes are primarily dependent on the dynamic interaction between the facilitator and participant.[8] Whether the participant perceived their relationship with the facilitator as positive or negative directly results in whether the participant feels psychologically safe in an SBE.[7] Stephen and colleagues[9] identified notable characteristics through their research that can provide key points in effectively creating psychologically safe environments (**Box 1**).

DISCUSSION

The concept of ethics is multidimensional, interfacing with almost every aspect of the world around us. Ethical decision-making and thought processes in healthcare occurs frequently require decision-making models and frameworks to "untangle" the complexities of ethical challenges in healthcare, especially in the ever-changing healthcare system with increasing patient diversity and complexities.[11] Without these ethical

---

Box 1
Key points to create a psychologically safe environment

- Create a supportive environment with positive verbal and nonverbal interactions.
- Establish a judgment-free learning environment where mistakes are ok and confidentiality is maintained.
- Foster respectful collaboration between the facilitator and students. Allow students to work together to solve problems.
- Clearly set expectations and explain what will occur during their simulation experience.
- Allow students a voice in discussing positive aspects of their experience. Frame opportunities for improvement within a positive learning context.
- Promote student confidence in their ability by focusing on learning opportunities and growth.[10]

Data from Stephen L-A, Kostovich C, O'Rourke J. Psychological Safety in Simulation: Prelicensure Nursing Students' Perceptions. Clin Sim. 2020;47:25-31. https://doi.org/10.1016/j.ecns.2020.06.010.

frameworks, clinicians are at risk of applying their personal moral compasses to ethical problem-solving situations, potentially violating the most basic tenant of patient care: do no harm.[10]

While no single model or framework applies to every situation, many models of ethical and moral thinking processes can be broadly applied to a variety of situations. There are subtle differences between the two, however, the concepts of "ethic" and "moral" are closely related. For the purposes of this discussion, these concepts are used interchangeably.

For learners and educators to prepare for SBEs that explore ethical and moral dilemmas in clinical practice, they must arm themselves with the knowledge of foundational ethical frameworks and models that will allow them to navigate difficult clinical decisions involving moral reasoning. Without the knowledge and skills necessary for creating effective solutions to ethical dilemmas, practicing nurses risk moral distress and burnout.[12] A primer on ethical frameworks follows with several important ethical frameworks and models that can be utilized both in preparation for the SBE and as a tool for navigating debriefing sessions involving ethical and moral patient care situations. Using these frameworks and models, educators can design scenarios and guided debriefing questions for a robust simulation experience. Students in turn will have a framework to establish moral competencies in their own professional nursing practice.

Western moral philosophy plays a critical role in the development of theoretic frameworks for moral and ethical conduct and decision-making. Steeped in the ethical theories of deontology and teleology (**Box 2**), 3 key ethical theories are important to consider: (1) ethical principles (ethical principlism); (2) moral rights (moral rights theory); and (3) moral virtues (virtue ethics).[10] Each of these theories is essential to consider as each has been developed in the context of practice and can be applied and revised depending on the situation.[10]

Ethical principlism is founded in the notion that the best ethical decisions are based on the moral principles of autonomy, nonmaleficence, beneficence, and justice[10] (**Box 3**). In an elegant explanation of ethical principlism, Johnstone[10] gives the example of making a measurement with a ruler. If the object being measured with a ruler is congruent with the desired length, the individual would judge the length as "correct." If the desired object is not congruent with the desired length as measured with the ruler, the individual would judge the length as "incorrect." In ethical principlism, if an ethical *action* "measures up" to the ethical *principle* (autonomy, nonmaleficence, beneficence, justice) we are measuring it against, the ethical action is considered "correct." If it does not, the ethical action is considered "incorrect."

Ethical Principlism in Simulation

When using ethical principlism, one must ponder the true foundational moral principles that should be used to "measure" our ethical actions and decide which moral

---

Box 2
The parent theories of deontology and teleology

Deontology (from the Greek deon, meaning "duty," and logos, meaning "word" or "reasoned discourse") prescribes some acts to be obligatory regardless of their consequences.

Teleology (from the Greek telos, meaning "end," and logos, meaning "word" or "reasoned discourse") prescribes some acts to be obligatory regardful of their consequences.

Data from Johnstone, M. Moral theory and the ethical practice of nursing. In: Bioethics: a nursing perspective. Chatswood, NSW: Churchill Livingstone Elsevier; 2023. p. 30-56.

Box 3
Summary of the 4 principles of ethical principlism

Autonomy—from the Greek autos (meaning "self") and nomos (meaning "rule," "governance," or "law"), literally "self-rule"; this principle stipulates that "persons should be respected as self-determining choosers"

Nonmaleficence—from the Latin-derived maleficent—from maleficus (meaning "wicked," "prone to evil"), from malum (meaning "evil"), and facere (meaning "to do"); this principle stipulates "do no harm"

Beneficence—from the Latin beneficus, from bene (meaning "well' or "good") and facere (meaning "to do"); this principle stipulates "above all, do good"

Justice—from Old Latin justus, from jus "law, right"; this principle primarily stipulates "do what is fair" (note that there are several interpretations of the notion of justice, which will be considered in further depth later in this section)

Data from Johnstone, M. Moral theory and the ethical practice of nursing. In: Bioethics: a nursing perspective. Chatswood, NSW: Churchill Livingstone Elsevier; 2023. p. 30-56.

---

principle(s) should be used in a particular situation.[10] Using ethical principlism as a foundational ethical theory, educators could formulate a simulation scenario involving a nurse who struggles with a family member's wishes to continue the patient's life support measures despite exhausting all treatments for a terminal illness. In the debrief session, the educator could refer to the principles of autonomy and nonmaleficence to guide the discussion and formulate recommendations with students regarding this complex patient scenario.

Theory of Moral Rights and Simulation

The theory of moral rights purports human beings have certain "rights" that must be morally and ethically protected.[10] These rights are not defined in a single list or definition but granted simply by being a human being (**Table 3**). Having a "right" to freedom or happiness, for example, is in and of itself enough to take a moral action.[10] Johnstone delineates 3 different types of moral rights: (1) inalienable rights that cannot be relegated to others; (2) absolute rights; and (3) prima facie rights that cannot be set aside by other moral claims.[10] The theory of moral rights can be challenging in situations where competing rights exist, when examining the connection between rights and responsibilities and ensuring all rights are equally considered.[10] Educators may choose to explore the theory of moral rights when discussing a simulation scenario in which a patient who is experiencing homelessness is being discharged from the hospital with a wound infection despite no plan for follow-up care with the provider. Does this situation intersect with certain moral rights we hold as human beings to access healthcare? What are the student's perspectives from the debrief session?

Dating back hundreds of years, virtue or character ethics continues to have a place in ethical frameworks important to today's ethical decision-making processes and thinking. Virtue ethics has a particular affinity for nursing as the virtuous nurse is equated with "the good nurse." The dilemma is defining what it means to be "virtuous."[10] For nursing, providing virtuous patient care (eg, care that is selfless, compassionate) is intertwined with the ethical care of the patient and the nurse–patient relationship.[10] Indeed, several national nursing organizations have ethical guidelines for patient care. Failing to provide ethical care may result in negative patient outcomes. Virtue ethics, such as ethical principlism and moral rights theories, is not without problems. Virtue theory does not delineate specific rules and definitions and thus is difficult to use when making

Table 3	
Simulation scenario examples of classic and contemporary theories of moral rights	
Classical and Contemporary Theories of Moral Rights	**What Would it Look Like in a Simulation Scenario?**
Moral rights based on natural law and divine command	Simulation Scenario: A patient refuses recommended medical care based on religious beliefs. How does the healthcare provider provide patient-centered care when the medical recommendation does not align with the religious beliefs?
Moral rights based on rationality	Simulation Scenario: There is a report of a family with significant injuries due to someone driving under the influence. Your patient is in the healthcare setting with significant wounds. During the scenario it is identified that the person receiving care is responsible for the accident and injuries of the family. How does the healthcare provider provide patient-centered care when the person has caused harm to others or gone against our moral code?
Moral rights based on special interests	Simulation Scenario: A patient is admitted to the hospital setting with a pet. He does not have a representative to take custody of the animal. As the primary nurse caring for the patient, how do you facilitate the situation?
Moral rights based on human experiences of grievous wrongs	Simulation Scenario: In an acute care facility, on a busy unit, during your shift you identify that a significant medication error has been made that causes harm to a patient. You realize that the error was made by another nurse on the unit and one of your closest colleagues and friends. Do you report the error and have your friend receive the negative consequence?

Data from Johnstone, M. Moral theory and the ethical practice of nursing. In: Bioethics: a nursing perspective. Chatswood, NSW: Churchill Livingstone Elsevier; 2023. p. 30-56.

an ethical decision.[10] In addition, what it takes to be a virtuous person often comes with expectations and demands that are unattainable.[10]

Models for Underpinning Simulation Scenarios

Outside of the ethical theoretic frameworks of ethical principlism, moral rights, and moral values, several models of ethical and moral thinking processes have emerged. Rest's model of moral action highlights the question: "What do we have to assume went on inside the head of a person who acts morally?"[13] **Table 4** outlines the 4 components of the model. All of the elements of the model are designed to be interactive, providing a pathway to the most common thinking process involved with moral and ethical decision-making. Failure to achieve any one of the elements of the model results in an inability to make an ethical/moral decision.[13,14] However, the Rest model stresses that there is no one right or wrong answer to an ethical dilemma. Rather, the elements of the model interact and have synergy with each other to produce an internal reaction that is congruent with acting morally in any given situation.[13,14] While this model could be the underpinnings for a specific self-guided reflection related to an ethical simulation scenario, it is approachable and easy-to-understand style could be adopted as a theoretic framework throughout an educational curriculum that discusses ethical situations that can be integrated into a controlled, simulation environment.

Table 4
Rest's model of moral action

Component	Description
I: Interpreting the situation	Acknowledging that the situation has ethical implications that could impact others
II: Formulating the morally ideal course of action	Exploring the situation and those involved to formulate options for next steps
III: Deciding what one actually intends to do	Acting in a way that prioritizes doing the right thing over being swayed by personal motivators
IV: Executing and implementing what one intends to do	Having the fortitude to carry out the moral action

From Rest, J.R. A psychologist looks at the teaching of ethics. The Hastings Center Report 1982; 12:29-36.

Recent contemporary models of ethical decision-making have been created using previous studies and qualitative approaches. These models serve as useful tools for educators when designing simulation scenarios and guided debriefing questions and provide useful frameworks for students as they develop their own moral competencies and decision-making skills. Park[11] designed an ethical decision-making model using information from a systematic literature review of 20 ethical decision-making models. In the literature review, which included articles applying the frameworks of ethical principlism, moral rights, and virtue theory to ethical decision-making, Park[11] found that while many of the models and theories had a similar clear stepwise approach to ethical decision-making, most of the models did not address or allow for consideration of the *context* of the ethical challenge.[11] By synthesizing these various models, Park[11] created a new, clinically practical model of integrated ethical decision-making. The model was subsequently piloted with baccalaureate nursing students in an ethics course.

The following 6 tenants of ethical decision-making are outlined in the model developed by Park[11]: (1) state the ethical problem; (2) collect additional information to analyze the problem; (3) develop alternatives and analyze and compare them; (4) select the best alternative and justify the decision; (5) develop strategies to successfully implement the chosen alternative and take action; and (6) evaluate the effects of the action and the decision-making process. Students in the pilot study reported that the model was easy to use and allowed for an increase in the number of options available for solving an ethical problem. The model also allowed students to make decisions based on rationale rather than intuition.[11]

Using a qualitative approach, Koskinen and colleagues[15] gathered ethical themes during conversations with scientific researchers and clinical practice providers resulting in the creation of an interdisciplinary ethical competence model. The model outlines 3 themes important to ethical practice: (1) ethical attitude to personally act in an ethical way; (2) ethical basis that has the patient's best interest at heart; and (3) ethical culture that values the common good.[15] The model is further supported by themes of having time to discuss and self-reflect with the healthcare team when making ethical decisions, and the importance of leadership in the sense of involving others outside of the team to acknowledge the larger organizational context.[15] While this model is in the early development stages, it is a good first step in understanding the team role in ethical decision-making and would be an ideal model to replicate in an interdisciplinary simulation scenario.

SUMMARY

Instilling moral reasoning skills is a vital competency necessary for optimal nursing care. Rooted in simulation-specific standards, ethics, and best practices, simulationists can create an inclusive, diverse, and psychologically safe environment ripe for acquisition of these crucial skills. When combined with the knowledge gained through ethical decision-making models and frameworks, learners can ultimately tap into their own consciousness when faced with moral and ethical dilemmas inherent in our healthcare system.

CLINICS CARE POINTS

- There are many important aspects in the development of simulation-based education; however, professional integrity and the practice of the Healthcare Simulationist Code of Ethics are the foundation to high-quality of simulation.

- Ethical expectations align professional nursing practice to simulation.

- Ethical expectations in simulation are applied to all involved in the simulation-based experience: learner, facilitator, and simulation operations specialist.

- More work is needed in the area of diversity, equity, inclusion, justice, and belonging within the realm of simulation.

DISCLOSURE

The authors have no commercial or financial conflicts of interest or any funding sources.

REFERENCES

1. Maxworthy JC, Palaganas JC, Epps CA, et al. Defining excellence in simulation programs. Philadelphia, PA: Lippincott Williams & Wilkins; 2022.
2. Society for Simulation in Healthcare. Healthcare simulationist code of ethics. 2018. Available at: http://www.ssih.org/Code-of-Ethics.
3. INACSL Standards Committee. Bowler F, Klein M and Wilford A. Healthcare Simulation Standards of Best Practice professional integrity, *Clin Sim*, 58, 2021, 45–48.
4. Lewis KL, Bohnert CA, Gammon WL, et al. The Association of Standardized Patient Educators (ASPE) Standards of Best Practice (SOBP). Adv Simul 2017;2:10.
5. American Nurses Association. Code of ethics for nurses with interpretive statements. Nursesbooks. org; 2015.
6. Cowperthwait A. NLN/Jeffries simulation framework for simulated participant methodology. Clinical Simulation in Nursing 2020;42:12–21.
7. Turner S, Harder N, Martin D, et al. Psychological safety in simulation: Perspectives of nursing students and faculty. Nurse Educ Today 2023;122. N.PAG-N.PAG.
8. Jeffries P. The NLN Jeffries simulation theory. Philedelphia, PA: Lippincott Williams & Wilkins; 2021.
9. Stephen L-A, Kostovich C, O'Rourke J. Psychological Safety in Simulation: Prelicensure Nursing Students' Perceptions. Clin Sim 2020;47:25–31.
10. Johnstone M. Moral theory and the ethical practice of nursing. In: Bioethics: a nursing perspective. Chatswood, NSW: Churchill Livingstone Elsevier; 2023. p. 30–56.
11. Park E-J. An integrated ethical decision-making model for nurses. Nurs Ethics 2012;19:139–59.

12. Shayestehfard M, Torabizadeh C, Gholamzadeh S, et al. Ethical Sensitivity in Nursing Students: Developing a Context–based Education. Electron J Gen Med 2020;17(2):em195.
13. Rest JR. A psychologist looks at the teaching of ethics. Hastings Cent Rep 1982; 12:29–36.
14. Grace P. Professional responsibility, nurses, and conscientious objection: A framework for ethical evaluation. Nurs Ethics 2023;0:0.
15. Koskinen C, Kaldestad K, Rossavik B, et al. Multi-professional ethical competence in healthcare - an ethical model. Nurs Ethics 2022;29:1003–13.

Considerations for Culturally Congruent Healthcare for Simulation in Bedside Clinical Practice

Desiree A. Díaz, PhD, FNP-BC, CNE, CHSE-A, ANEF, FSSH, FAAN[a],*,
Valerie C. Martínez, DNP, APRN, CPNP-PC, PMHS[a],
Humberto López Castillo, MD, PhD, CPH, CMI-Spanish[b,c]

KEYWORDS

- Culturally congruent care • Simulation-based education • Health promotion
- Simulation applications • Best practices • Simulation design

KEY POINTS

- Culturally congruent practice is the individualized provision of health services that is sensitive and responsive to the cultural beliefs, values, and health practices of the patient.
- Cultural humility posits that a healthcare provider may not fully understand a patient's culture or practices but is willing to learn.
- Healthcare simulation-based education can implement culturally appropriate and congruent scenarios for learners, framed within cultural humility.
- The 11 criteria for simulation design outlined in the Healthcare Simulation Standards of Best Practice allow educators to prepare simulations.

INTRODUCTION

Nurses have cared for patients from diverse cultural backgrounds in the community setting for centuries.[1] The influence of culture on human health and health practices[2–4]

Disclaimer: The example provided in this article was funded through a grant from the Health Resources and Services Administration at the US Department of Health and Human Services (6 U4EHP46217-01-01).
^a Department of Nursing Practice, College of Nursing, Academic Health Sciences Center, University of Central Florida, Orlando, FL, USA; ^b Department of Health Sciences, College of Health Professions and Sciences, Academic Health Sciences Center, University of Central Florida, Orlando, FL, USA; ^c Department of Population Health Sciences, College of Medicine, Academic Health Sciences Center, University of Central Florida, Orlando, FL, USA
* Corresponding author. 12201 Research Parkway, Suite 300, Orlando, FL 32826.
E-mail address: desiree.diaz@ucf.edu

highlights the need for nurses and other healthcare providers to deliver culturally congruent healthcare. In 2015, the American Nurses Association added *culturally congruent practice* to nursing's Standards of Professional Performance.[5] Culturally congruent practice refers to individualized provision of health services that is sensitive and responsive to the cultural beliefs, values, and health practices of the patient.[5–7] The provision of health is further recognized by the World Health Organization as identifying the social and political constructs, specifically language access or barriers that can affect care.[7]

To effectively deliver culturally congruent healthcare, nurses and other healthcare providers need to approach care provision with a sense of cultural humility. Cultural humility identifies that a provider may not fully understand a patient's culture or practices but is willing to learn.[8] Exposure to clinical cultural training opportunities, for example, through simulation-based experiences (SBEs), is one effective way to help cultivate a sense of cultural humility.[9] Further, training in clinical cultural applications has demonstrated the potential for improved communication between providers and ethnic minority patients and the ability to overcome other barriers to care and disparities.[10] Unfortunately, there is a dearth of studies that specifically incorporate simulation best practices and reporting standards when developing and implementing cultural healthcare SBE training.[11]

Aim

The aim of this article is to provide practical recommendations for creating and implementing culturally appropriate[12] and culturally congruent[5] healthcare simulation applications for bedside providers that adhere to best practices and reporting standards.

Operational Definition

In the remainder of the article, we will utilize the unifying term of culturally congruent healthcare. Cultural congruence will encompass the totality of cultural appropriateness, cultural humility, cultural competence, and cultural sensitivity in an effort to discuss the topic broadly.

Design of the Healthcare Simulation Standards of Best Practice

This article will focus on the Healthcare Simulation Standards of Best Practice™ (HSSOBP™) simulation design, which provide 11 essential criteria for creating and designing culturally congruent healthcare simulations.[13] Each criterion and its rationale will be discussed, and practical examples of their application will be provided, framed within a scenario that involved Spanish-speaking farm workers. The scenario was funded by a Health Resources and Services Administration grant and has been published elsewhere.[14] Briefly, the simulation developed a scenario that explored healthcare disparities related to a migrant farm worker community. The scenario uses a public health framework to explore risk factors related to cardiovascular health and language access while investigating health promotion practices. Effectively incorporating the HSSOBP™ criteria can result in a well-crafted simulation scenario that can positively impact patient care.[14] The description of these 11 criteria, along with their summary and corresponding examples, is summarized in **Table 1**.

Criterion 1

SBEs should be vetted by experts in both the clinical content and the application of simulation for teaching purposes. The elements of the scenario should be informed

Table 1
Summary of the 11 International Nursing Association for Clinical Simulation and Learning essential criteria[13] for creating and designing culturally congruent healthcare simulations with the corresponding Health Resources and Services Administration example[14]

Criteria	Summary	Application/Example
1. The SBE should be vetted by clinical and simulation experts	• Clinical SMEs provide elements informed by EBP • Simulation SMEs provide elements reflecting current practices promoting optimal health outcomes	• Derive potential simulation scenarios from sentinel events at the clinic, hospital, or outpatient settings
2. Assess educational needs that can be addressed through SBE	• Identify educational needs prone to be addressed through simulation scenarios • Collect information from multiple sources: learners, clinicians, educators, outcome data, and practice guidelines	• Assessment of community resources in the primary language of the patient population, triangulated with clinic and ED providers • Verify learner's beliefs and attitudes toward the care of the patient population
3. Develop measurable, realistic objectives to guide the SBE	• Clear, measurable, realistic objectives that focus on and direct the background and case • Objectives will outline knowledge, skills, or behaviors that should be achieved	• Specific, measurable, attainable, realistic, and timed (SMART) objectives can be developed using the CDC guidance[14] • To recognize the difference between heat stroke and acute stroke by the end of the SBE
4. Ensure the SBE modality supports the SBE objectives	• Consider technology and equipment availability, focusing on the clinical setting • Type of simulation patient consideration (eg, mannequin, standardized patient, computer-based scenarios) • Specific skills needed for the task (eg, psychomotor, communication, or decision-making)	• Use the free clinic as a simulation scenario, after considering patient flow for regular activities • Equipment and surroundings mimic the clinic's reality, allowing the learner to create reference points for future applications
5. The scenario should establish the setting and context for the SBE	• Using real patients and scenarios in the clinic can serve as a backstory • Learners can relate to their patient population and environment	• In situ scenario at the free clinic 1 hour prior to patient arrival would provide an opportunity for learning without interfering with patient care
6. Creating realism is essential in the education of healthcare providers	• Auditory, visual, and kinesthetic cues create a relatable environment for the healthcare provider	• In the scenario, forms and charts actually in use at the free clinic were implemented as part of the learning experience • This ensures a relatable environment

(continued on next page)

Table 1
(continued)

Criteria	Summary	Application/Example
7. Implementation of the SBE for all learners should be carefully planned	• Planning incorporates the facilitator (eg, learning objectives, subject matter expertise, skills), the scenario (eg, materials, flow), and the learners (eg, readings to complete before the SBE)	• Facilitators without SME trained on specific skills and procedures before the SBE, so they can convey the basics to the learners • However, SMEs were available in case learners required additional feedback beyond the skills provided by the trained facilitator
8. Prebrief materials allow learners to understand expectations for the SBE	• Expectations are important for adult learners for optimal success	• Primary care providers were prebriefed about medications available for prescription and its indications • A structured report, intake sheet, and information about the patient were also prebriefed to the clinicians guiding the SBE
9. The debrief, reflection, and feedback phase requires proper attention	• It is key to understand the learner group and the environment where the SBE took place • Proper planning of the feedback should consider alternative scenarios or pathways ("what-if's")	• Debriefing allowed to reiterate linguistic barriers, given that the population in the SBE (and in the clinic) primarily speaks Spanish • Adequate discussion of caring for populations with LEP
10. Evaluation strategies respond to the learning objectives and is planned before implementing the SBE	• Formal and informal and summative or formative evaluations can be implemented based on the learning objectives • Learners should be aware of both the learning objectives and the evaluation strategies before entering the SBE	• Informal, formative evaluation: A simple checklist with criteria to request an interpreter for people with LEP and proper prescription management • Formal, summative evaluation: Can repeat the previous steps, with the learner aware of performance expectations
11. Pilot-testing is fundamental to further develop the SBE	• Both instructors and learners can contribute to enriching the SBE after running a pilot of the scenario • Nuances and potential difficulties of the SBE can be addressed beforehand	• A group of providers and nurses pilot-tested the intraprofessional scenario in the clinic • Monitorization of timing, patient flow, and resource utilization allowed for a successful SBE

Abbreviations: CDC, Centers for Disease Control and Prevention; EBP, evidence-based practice; ED, emergency department; LEP, limited English proficiency; SBE, simulation-based experience; SME, subject matter expert.

by evidence-based practices and reflect current practices that promote optimal health outcomes. The background content of the scenario is only half of the needed expertise to create a phenomenal learning environment. Engaging simulation experts to review the SBE is beneficial. An expert can be identified through credentials such as Certified Healthcare Simulation Educator (CHSE). CHSE-prepared faculty are knowledgeable of the principles of adult learning and the effective use of technology in simulation-based learning experiences.

Rationale. Clinicians of all types have various expertise related to patient care. However, clinical expertise alone does not necessarily translate into effective education practices. SBE is a specialty that has been extensively researched and can be extremely beneficial for learners. The distinct value of combining both clinical and simulation expertise when developing a culturally congruent healthcare simulation can create a catalyst for improved patient outcomes by providing impactful education experiences for learners.

Application/example. A sentinel event can take place in the clinic, hospital, and/or an outpatient setting. Utilizing the actual events to create a simulation scenario can offer 2 benefits, one of learning from a major event and the other of preventing future situations. It is still a necessity to utilize simulation experts to validate the technical and educational components of the scenario to ensure simulation effectiveness.

Criterion 2
Conducting a needs assessment to identify educational needs that can be addressed through appropriate simulation scenarios is essential for proper planning. The needs assessment should involve gathering information from multiple sources, including learners, clinicians, educators, outcome data, and practice guidelines. It is important to establish whom the scenario is to benefit, and then seek input from those stakeholders.

Rationale. This criterion is grounded in the principle that the learners involved in the education need to feel the information is valuable based on adult learning principles.[15] Additionally, it is important to provide learning opportunities that address relevant competencies based on stakeholder needs.

Application/example. The community in which the clinic was associated had a large migrant farm worker population and the primary language of that particular group was Spanish. Seeking information from the community resources services that provide information to the population as well as the community leaders helped guide the creation of a scenario based on what they feel is needed for the community.[14] This was then triangulated with providers that care for the farm workers in the clinic or emergency rooms. Further, seeking information on learner beliefs and attitudes surrounding caring for this patient population can provide valuable information for the design of the scenario.

Criterion 3
The creation of objectives is key when designing an evidence-based scenario. Objectives that are measurable and realistic should be constructed following HSSOBP™ objectives and outcomes.[16] These objectives guide the specific aspects that need to be included in the background and case.

Rationale. This criterion ensures that there is a clear focus and direction for the simulation by outlining the specific knowledge, skills, or behaviors that learners should achieve by the end of the simulation. Objectives serve as a basis for communicating the expectations of the scenario to the learners and for evaluating the effectiveness of the simulation experience.

Application/example. Nursing-specific, measurable, attainable, realistic, and timed (SMART) objectives were created for the public health scenario.[17] One of the SMART objectives was to "recognize the difference between heat stroke and acute stroke (specific) by the end of the SBE (timed). The main difference between heat stroke (flushed/red skin, rapid shallow breathing) and cardiovascular stroke is the presence of facial droop and inability to have laterality when smiling or arm weakness (measurable)."[14] This objective was attainable and realistic for the specified time frame.

Criterion 4

Creating the ultimate scenario includes considering where and how the SBE will be conducted to ensure the chosen modality supports the simulation objectives. The use of technology and the availability of equipment need to be considered. SBE for healthcare providers can be conducted in situ, directly in the clinical setting[18] or in a simulated setting in a learning laboratory. If the SBE will take place on the unit or in the clinic environment, considerations should be made regarding the timing of the simulation and the patient flow within the clinic or unit. The safety of actual patients in an in- situ environment needs to be given the utmost priority. Additionally, considerations regarding the type of simulation patient used may include options such a static mannequin, standardized patient, or computer-based scenarios. Finally, it is important to consider whether there are specific skills associated with the SBE that need to be incorporated in the design. This may involve psychomotor tasks, communication skills, or decision-making processes that are essential for the targeted learning objectives.

Rationale. Identifying how the scenario will be portrayed within the context of the SBE will create a cohesive and effective learning experience. If the scenario is in a pop-up free clinic, the environment should reflect this. The equipment and surroundings should mimic the reality of having a clinic in the field. Creating realism will allow the learner to create reference points for future applications.

Application/example. The public health scenario is set in a simulated free clinic. This free clinic replicated the actual setting rather than in situ.

Criterion 5

The scenario should be created in a way that establishes the setting and context for the SBE. Utilizing current real-patient scenarios that have occurred in the clinic or at the bedside can be the inspiration for the backstory of the scenario. This offers a rich experience as learners are familiar with their standard clientele and patient population. Additionally, each scenario should identify critical actions that learners are required to complete in order to achieve the scenario objectives.

Rationale. Offering a backstory provides learners with a realistic starting point for the SBE. Critical actions facilitate the progression of learners in the scenario toward achievement of the SBE objectives and provide an evaluation measure of learner performance. Providing scripted context for the scenario also ensures consistency and standardization, which contributes to the validity and reliability of the scenario.

Application/example. If the educators wanted to create an in situ SBE, use of the clinic space an hour prior to patient arrival can be an opportunity for a rich learning environment. The in situ scenario would not interfere with patient care and would minimize the need to obtain extra props.

Criterion 6

Creating realism is essential in the education of healthcare providers. This can be achieved within an SBE by employing different types of fidelity. Auditory, visual, and kinesthetic cues associated with the scenario can create an environment the provider and the learner can relate to.

Rationale. Relatability is fundamental and the cues within the SBE should convey a familiar, relatable case where learners can build from prior experiences within the environment and associate it with new cues. Using different forms of fidelity helps to maximize the relatability and realism of the scenario for the learner.

Application/example. In a free clinic, having the most up-to-date electronic health record may not be realistic. In this case, using what was actually found in the clinic created a level of realism that elevated the SBE to a more realistic immersive environment. In this scenario, thus, we implemented paper forms and charts that simulate the everyday operational environment in the free clinic, along with examination rooms and patient flow algorithms that, although not high-tech, still conveyed high fidelity to everyday scenarios.

Criterion 7

The implementation of the SBE for all learners should be thoroughly planned. This includes preparing learners using required reading prior to participating in the SBE, facilitating the scenario, and conducting a comprehensive debriefing session afterward. Crucial elements to planning include proper training and professional development for the facilitator responsible for conducting the SBE, particularly as it relates to the incorporation of culturally appropriate and congruent care.

Rationale. A facilitator who is not a subject matter expert (SME) can conduct certain SBEs, but they cannot replace the importance of having someone with the subject matter expertise involved in the SBE.[19] For example, if a nurse is the facilitator, they may not be able to effectively guide students through the proper steps of a specific skill or procedure. In this case, the nurse facilitator can be taught by the SME; however, additional resources should be available as needed by the learners, based on the objectives of the SBE.

Application/example. In the public health scenario example, a SME guided the simulation facilitator prior to the delivery of the SBE. A public health nurse with experience practicing in a free migrant clinic, who was also trained in simulation-based pedagogy, was utilized to guide students through the SBE.

Criterion 8

An important element of the SBE is the prebrief material that students engage with before participating in the SBE. Having required prebrief material allows learners to be fully prepared prior to the start of the SBE. The prebrief allows the learners to understand the dynamics of the SBE and what is required.

Rationale. Developing a prebriefing plan helps to adequately prepare learners for the SBE. The prebrief plan ensures that clear expectations are set before the scenario begins. Clearly defined expectations are important for adult learners to achieve optimal success in the SBE.

Application/example. Before participating in an SBE, clinicians may need to receive new protocols or procedures prior to the SBE. This information can be provided in the form of an article or algorithm that aligns with the learning objectives. In the public health scenario, the primary care provider is working at the free health clinic via telehealth. Details of the medication that was available for prescribing was provided to learners as prebrief material. Additionally, during the prebrief, or immediate time prior to the SBE, a report was given to the learner about the patient.[18] The report was a structured intake sheet with relevant information pertaining to the case. Prebrief material also included telehealth etiquette, interprofessional strategies, and culturally congruent care initiatives.

Criterion 9
The debriefing or reflection and feedback phase is an aspect of the SBE that requires proper attention. Understanding the learner group and the environment in which the discussion is going to take place will improve the effectiveness of the SBE. Properly planning the feedback process should incorporate consideration of potential "what if" scenarios to ensure a comprehensive debriefing experience.

Rationale. Creating a space in which learners can explore their feelings and thinking requires proper planning.

Application/example. Debriefing the clinician caring for the farm worker included linguistic care and appropriate telehealth actions. Regardless of whether it was identified in the objectives, knowing that the population primarily speaks Spanish necessitates a discussion on proper care for people with limited English proficiency, including the use of Culturally and Linguistically Appropriate Services standards.[12]

Criterion 10
Evaluation of the learners should be based on the objectives and decided during the creation of the SBE. Learners should be aware before the start of the SBE. Evaluation can be informal or formal, as well as formative or summative.

Application/example. Informal evaluation of the farm workers' clinic could include a simple checklist on requesting an interpreter and proper prescription management based on the new formulary. Formal evaluation can be the same 2 assessments; however, there may be a consequence regarding performance.

Criterion 11
Pilot testing is a fantastic way to figure out what needs further development. Having a learner or 2 participate in the SBE prior to the implementation of the scenario with learners can create a more realistic environment as the nuances are corrected.

Rationale. Understanding the nuances of an SBE prior to learner engagement provides optimal learning. Educators who have deliberately taken the time to work through problems with scenario design have improved outcomes.[20]

Application/example. The farmworker scenario was pilot-tested with a group of undergraduate learners, registered nurses, and practicing providers. Further exploration can be conducted to increase the number of participants in the intraprofessional scenario. This would take place in the in situ clinic 1 hour beforehand. The timing and patient flow would be monitored to ensure optimal utilization of time and resources prior to the transition with all participants/learners.

DISCUSSION

In this article, we address the importance of cultural congruence in healthcare SBEs for learners with rational and direct applications. There has been limited representation in reported SBE.[21–24] The content infused in a properly designed simulation has the natural tendency to create deliberate objectives around providing culturally congruent care and eliminating healthcare discrepancies.

A framework to initiate the work of cultural congruence designed in scenarios is needed to ensure best practices. The potential infusion of biases must be mitigated and can be limited when adhering to structured guidelines. This article offers some "take-home" applications that allow the educator to immediately implement in a scenario with cultural content. The key is to have clear objectives with deliberate messaging from the prebrief to the completion of the debrief.

Future applications and directions need to be focused on encouraging providers to create, test, and report findings on implementing provocative content within the curricula at the practice level. Translation to practice is the next step that is needed to ensure patients begin receiving the care they need and deserve regardless of status.

CLINICS CARE POINTS

- Culturally congruent care and cultural humility require incorporating diversity in simulation-based education.
- When designing simulation-based education scenarios, the HSSOBP™ present an excellent implementation and evaluation framework.

DISCLOSURE

The authors have no financial disclosures relevant to this publication.

REFERENCES

1. Seacole M. Wonderful adventures of Mrs. Seacole in many lands. London, England: James Blackwood; 1857.
2. Giger JN, Haddad L. Transcultural nursing: Assessment and intervention. 8th edition. St. Louis, MO: Elsevier; 2021.
3. McFarland MR, Wehbe-Alamah HB. Leininger's culture care diversity and universality: A worldwide nursing theory. 3rd edition. Sudbury, MA: Jones and Bartlett Learning; 2015.
4. Schim SM, Doorenbos AZ. A three-dimensional model of cultural congruence: Framework for intervention. J Soc Work End Life Palliat Care 2010;6(3–4): 256–70.
5. Hegge M, Fowler M, Bjarnason D, et al. Code of ethics for nurses with interpretive statements. 2nd edition. Silver Spring, MD: American Nurses Association; 2015.
6. Marion L, Douglas M, Lavin MA, et al. Implementing the new ANA Standard 8: Culturally congruent practice. Online J Issues Nurs 2016;22(1):9.
7. World Health Organization. WHO recommends considering cultural factors to develop more inclusive health systems. 2020. https://www.who.int/news-room/

feature-stories/detail/who-recommends-considering-cultural-factors-to-develop-more-inclusive-health-systems. [Accessed 22 December 2023].

8. Foronda C. A theory of cultural humility. J Transcult Nurs 2020;31(1):7–12.

9. Hughes V, Delva S, Nkimbeng M, et al. Not missing the opportunity: Strategies to promote cultural humility among future nursing faculty. J Prof Nurs 2020;36(1): 28–33.

10. Suurmond J, Lieveld A, van de Wetering M, et al. Towards culturally competent paediatric oncology care. A qualitative study from the perspective of care providers. Eur J Cancer Care 2017;26(6). https://doi.org/10.1111/ecc.12680.

11. Walsche N, Condon C, Gonzales RA, et al. Cultural simulations, authenticity, focus, and outcomes: A systematic review of the healthcare literature. Clin Simul Nurs 2022;71:65–81.

12. US Department of Health and Human Services. Office of Minority Health. National Standards for Culturally and Linguistically Appropriate Services (CLAS) in Health and Health Care. https://thinkculturalhealth.hhs.gov/assets/pdfs/Enhanced NationalCLASStandards.pdf. [Accessed 22 December 2023].

13. INACSL Standards Committee, Watts PI, McDermott DS, Alinier G, et al. Healthcare Simulation Standards of Best Practice™ Simulation Design. Clin Simul Nurs 2021;58:14–21.

14. Díaz DA, Anderson M, Guido-Sanz F, Hill P, Spears S. The iING's of Public Health Scenarios (PHS), creating, validating, assessing. Health Resources and Services Administration (HRSA) of the U.S. Department of Health and Human Services (HHS) grant number 6 U4EHP46217-01-01, Public Health Simulation-Infused Program (PHSIP). Poster presented at: International Nursing Association of Clinical Simulation and Learning (INACSL), Providence, RI.

15. Mezirow J. A critical theory of adult learning and education. In: Tight M, editor. Education for adults. London, England: Routledge; 1983. https://doi.org/10.4324/ 9780203802670.

16. INACSL Standards Committee, Miller C, Deckers C, Jones M, et al. Healthcare Simulation Standards of Best Practice™ Outcomes and Objectives. Clin Simul Nurs 2021;58:40–4.

17. Centers for Disease Control and Prevention, *Writing SMART objectives. Evaluation briefs*, 2018, 3b. 2018. Available at: https://www.cdc.gov/healthyyouth/ evaluation/pdf/brief3b.pdf. Accessed December 23, 2023.

18. Lioce L (Ed.), Lopreiato J (Founding Ed.), Downing D, Chang TP, Robertson JM, Anderson M, Díaz DA, Spain AE (Assoc. eds); Terminology and Concepts Working Group. Healthcare simulation dictionary, 2.1 ed. Agency for Healthcare Research and Quality; September 2020. AHRQ Publication No. 20-0019. doi:10.23970/simulationv2.

19. Díaz DA, Gonzalez L, Anderson M, et al. Implications of subject matter expertise as a requirement for debriefing: A randomized control trial. Simulat Gaming 2020; 51(6):770–84.

20. Anderson M, Campbell S, Nye C, et al. Simulation in advanced practice education: Let's dialogue. Clin Simul Nurs 2019;26:81–5.

21. Díaz DA, Murillo CL, Bryant K, et al. The use of racial and ethnic healthcare disparities in simulation-based experiences: A systematic review. Clin Simul Nurs 2023;83:101440.

22. Díaz DA, Todd A, Gilbert GE, et al. Using various types of embedded participants to enhance culturally congruent, family-centered simulation-based education. Simulat Gaming 2023;54(4):427–46.

23. Murillo CL, Díaz DA, Tamanna N, et al. Social determinants of health in graduate nursing simulation education: An integrative review. Nurse Educat 2023. https://doi.org/10.1097/NNE.0000000000001561.
24. Smallheer B, Chidume T, Spinks MKH, et al. A scoping review of the priority of diversity, inclusion, and equity in healthcare simulation. Clin Simul Nurs 2022; 71:41–64.

Setting Learners up for Simulation and Clinical Success: Achieving Psychological Safety

Donna S. McDermott, PhD, RN, CHSE-A[a],*,
Samantha Smeltzer, DNP, RN, CHSE[b],
Jessica L. Kamerer, EdD, MSN, RNC-NIC[c]

KEYWORDS

- Prebriefing • Clinical practice • Nursing • Psychological safety • Briefing
- Competency • Continuing education

KEY POINTS

- Healthcare settings require continuing education and competency demonstration for both new and experienced registered nurses. Simulation is an effective method to use for teaching and competency demonstration but requires special skills and training.
- The International Nursing Association for Clinical Simulation and Learning developed standards of best practice in simulation as a guide to use simulation for teaching, learning, and evaluating competency in clinical practice.
- Promoting a psychologically safe learning and practice environment for new and experienced nurses assists with decreasing anxiety and creates a safe workplace environment.

INTRODUCTION/BACKGROUND

Owing to fast-paced working environments, increased patient acuity, nursing shortages, and new technologies, healthcare settings present challenges for both new and experienced registered nurses. Continuing education and competency demonstration are essential for keeping up with these demands of the nursing profession. Often used in the nursing academic setting, simulation can also be an effective method for learning and demonstrating competency in the clinical setting. Simulation has value in helping all clinicians acquire new knowledge, skills, and attitudes in

[a] University of South Florida College of Nursing, 12901 Bruce B. Downs Boulevard, Tampa FL 33612, USA; [b] Orbis Education, 301 North Pennsylvania Parkway, Suite 400 Indianapolis, IN 46032, USA; [c] Corporate Programs & Lifetime Learning, Center for Innovative Teaching, Nursing, Robert Morris University, 6001 University Boulevard, Moon Twp, PA 15108, USA
* Corresponding author.
E-mail address: donnamcdermott@usf.edu

Nurs Clin N Am 59 (2024) 383–390
https://doi.org/10.1016/j.cnur.2024.02.004
0029-6465/24/© 2024 Elsevier Inc. All rights reserved.

nursing.theclinics.com

testing new and existing care environments for latent safety risks and transitioning newly licensed registered nurses from student to professional roles.[1] Clinical settings for these types of simulation use can include, but are not limited to, acute care hospitals, long-term care facilities, outpatient clinics or care centers, and urgent care units.

Most newly licensed nurses have had simulation experiences during their education and may expect it as part of their ongoing professional development throughout their careers.[1] In 2018, the Association for Nursing Professional Development, the Society of Simulation in Healthcare Nursing Section, and the International Nursing Association for Clinical Simulation and Learning (INACSL) investigated the use of simulation in transition-to-practice (TTP) programs. Through literature review, the organizations sought to identify how simulation was used to support newly graduated nurses within their first 6 to 12 months after hire in their first nursing positions. The goal for TTP was to help them move from functioning in the role of a student to being competent, functional professional nurses.[2] TTP programs can include programs such as graduate nurse orientation and nurse residency programs. TTP programs are commonly used in hospitals and acute care settings and employ nurse educators or nursing professional development departments to plan, coordinate, and facilitate simulation. Simulation can be conducted in a separate simulation setting or also in situ (within the actual patient care environments) in real clinical settings.

Just as nurses are familiar with using patient care guidelines and standards to inform their clinical practices, simulation educators also have standards of best practice to guide their use of simulation for teaching, learning, and evaluating competencies. One of these standards, prebriefing, discusses how to prepare learners and how to create a psychologically safe learning environment during simulation. This article assists clinical educators in the application of this standard of best practice to create a prebriefing plan and prepare learners for simulation in the clinical setting. In addition, these concepts will be used to demonstrate how they can be applied beyond the simulation setting to clinical practice.

THE HEALTHCARE SIMULATION STANDARDS OF BEST PRACTICE

The INACSL developed the initial set of simulation standards of best practice in 2011. Since that time, simulation education has evolved through research and practice. In 2021, the INACSL Standards were revised and rebranded to the Healthcare Simulation Standards of Best Practice (HSSOBP™)[3] and included 2 new simulation standards.[3] One of the newer standards added was the HSSOBP™ Prebriefing: Preparation and Briefing.[4] Prebriefing is the process of preparing simulation participants for the simulation experience (**Fig. 1**). Elements of this standard include ensuring learners have the knowledge to participate, setting the rules of engagement, and establishing a safe learning environment. The Prebriefing HSSOBP™ emphasizes that the simulation facilitator and developer should be knowledgeable about the scenario and competent in simulation and prebriefing best practices.[4] According to this Prebriefing standard, consideration of the learner and the learning objectives is the driving force behind development of the prebriefing plan.[4] Another aspect of the standard is the establishment of a psychologically safe learning environment during the prebriefing.[4,5] A psychologically safe learning environment can be achieved by the educator taking time to explain the simulation logistics, the expectations for participation (including any evaluation methods), and setting the tone for a trusting learning environment that encourages risk-free decision-making. In addition, the simulation educator should inform learners that there will be an opportunity for reflective debriefing after the simulation.

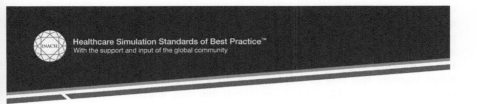

PREBRIEFING: PREPARATION AND BRIEFING

Criteria Necessary to Meet this Standard:

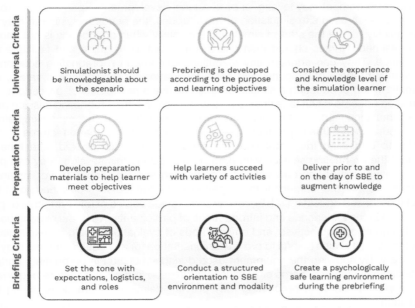

Universal Criteria

Simulationist should be knowledgeable about the scenario

Prebriefing is developed according to the purpose and learning objectives

Consider the experience and knowledge level of the simulation learner

Preparation Criteria

Develop preparation materials to help learner meet objectives

Help learners succeed with variety of activities

Deliver prior to and on the day of SBE to augment knowledge

Briefing Criteria

Set the tone with expectations, logistics, and roles

Conduct a structured orientation to SBE environment and modality

Create a psychologically safe learning environment during the prebriefing

Fig. 1. Prebriefing: Preparation and Briefing Standard Simofographic. (2021 INACSL. Used with permission.)

Simulation Prebriefing

Nurses who are designing simulation for clinical practice areas such as nurse residency programs, clinical competency evaluation, or professional development experiences need to balance the need for a realistic, meaningful, and challenging learning experience with the necessity to maintain the psychological safety of their learners. Clinical nurse educators must also recognize each new hire brings a different level of skills and experience that can also cause psychological safety imbalance. Utilization of the HSSOBP™ Prebriefing standard enables nurses to find this balance.[4]

Psychological safety has been defined as a *"shared belief that the team is safe for interpersonal risk-taking."*[6] Interpersonal risks, in the context of simulation learning, may include voicing concerns, asking questions, performing in simulation, and seeking feedback. In psychologically safe simulations, participants can do perform without fear of reprimand, judgment, or loss of peer/supervisor respect. To thoroughly engage in the simulation activity, learners must feel safe to try new methods of practice or thinking, experiment, ask questions, make mistakes, and receive feedback. When learners feel free to fully engage, they have a richer and more meaningful learning experience. One way to establish this safe environment for learning is to create a prebriefing plan.

The first step in the prebriefing plan is to identify the target learners and their levels of expertise. Nurses planning simulation can do this prior to the time of implementation. For example, TTP simulation outcomes and expectations for newly hired registered nurses (RNs) may look very different than experiences for nurses with multiple years of experience. Hospital educators and mentors should anticipate performing a quick needs assessment of their new nurses to determine their current level of skills and knowledge. This needs assessment can be done in preplanning for programming such as TTP, competency testing, or professional development experiences. In some instances, such as in situ simulation or mock codes, the needs assessment may be done quickly before the start of simulation especially when attendance is not known or preplanned. Nurses should then use this information to guide and facilitate the experience. They can address any identified concerns in a prebriefing session to adequately prepare participants and set a foundation for psychological safety. For example, when conducting a simulation that will use a new policy or procedure, the simulation educators can take time to review the policy in the prebriefing session prior to the simulation start. Or, if participants have not used the simulation manikin before, they should spend time in prebriefing reviewing the functionality and features.

Prior to beginning the simulation, the simulation educator should take time to conduct the prebriefing session with participants. During this session, they can provide explanations of key concepts of a prebriefing session (**Table 1**). For instance, items to prepare the learner for the experience are the logistics or schedule of the simulation-based education (SBE), review and provide copies of any protocols or policies used in the experience and introductions of participants. Next, the expectations, learning goals and objectives, and any methods of evaluation should be explained.

At this time, it is also helpful to provide an orientation for any equipment that may be necessary. By showing the equipment used during simulation in prebriefing, participants can have their concerns or questions addressed immediately before beginning. An equipment review in prebriefing may prevent delays or distractions during the simulation.

Lastly, the simulation educators should share the purpose of the session and explain the concepts of a safe learning environment and psychological safety. Emphasis on simulation for the purposes of learning and feedback rather than punishment or ridicule is essential. Telling simulation learners to participate the best of their knowledge and capabilities serves as a reminder that simulation is a method for learning and reinforcing skills. Simulation educators who provide these details will help decrease anxiety and stress for learners during the simulation.

Prebriefing Beyond the Simulation Environment

Delivering prebriefing to professional nurses in the clinical setting is not as novel as one may assume. Incorporating elements of best practice from the HSSOBP™: Prebriefing can be seen as a strategic approach in leadership positions, such as charge nurse, preceptors, and mentors.[4] Just as simulation educators use the HSSOBP™ standard to "set the stage" for learners, clinical nurse educators can also achieve

Table 1
Applying prebriefing concepts to the clinical setting

HSSOBP™ Prebriefing Concepts	Simulation Prebriefing Plan for TTP, Nurse Residency, and In Situ Simulations	Prebriefing Strategies for Application to the Clinical Setting
Reflect on your own level of expertise and competency	Have you facilitated simulation before? How comfortable are you with simulation teaching and learning? Do you have any professional development needs to ensure you are using best practices in simulation education?	Have you precepted new nurses or students? How comfortable are you with precepting or orienting new nurses? What learning needs do you have to serve as a preceptor or mentor or nursing leader?
Assess the learner	Needs assessment of current level of expertise and knowledge	Needs assessment of level of nursing skill and knowledge
Prepare the learner	Review skills to be used in the simulation. Provide copies of treatment protocols or guidelines. Consider a written prebriefing plan to standardize the simulation for all learners.	Provide copies of treatment protocols or guidelines. Introduce new nurses to unit personnel and team. Identify areas for improvement and further development.
Clarify goals and learning objectives	Review the purpose and learning objectives of the simulation	Perform daily huddles where nursing leaders' brief team. Deliver patient goal-oriented report to provide new nurses with strategies for patient care.
Create a psychologically safe learning environment	Provide logistics of the day. Review the simulation expectations and roles of participants. Demonstrate methods of communication during simulation. Support risk taking during simulation to challenge learners.	Allow new nurses to ask questions. Provide orientation and clarification. Provide direct and immediate feedback. Set expectations. Include interprofessional teams. Seek input and encourage new ideas. Treat team members with respect. Foster an environment of integrity and trust. Prevent defensive behavior.
Orient to equipment and technology	Review simulation room and equipment. Allow time to explore manikins and other equipment. Explain what can and cannot be simulated.	Orient to the clinical environment. Provide new equipment training

this in the clinical setting. By following the core elements of prebriefing, nurse leaders can prepare nurses to provide a safe environment prior to their shift (see **Fig. 1**). Allowing a new orienteer to feel safe in the beginning stages of the orientation period may provide comfort and lead to a better mental space to learn new processes.

In addition, providing a safe space can allow the nurses to mentally prepare for the workday, provide an opportunity for reflection and anticipation of the clinical day. Additionally for mentors and preceptors, prebriefing before the clinical day allows clarification of assignments, review of the goals for the day, enhances novice nurses' confidence, and allows application of theory into practice.

Some applications for using elements of the prebriefing standards of best practice (SOBP) in the hospital setting include.

1. Clarify goals and learning objectives

During briefing, nurse leaders can clearly articulate goals of the day, ensuring that nurses understand what they are expected to achieve. The goals can be aligned to professional development or orientation training. The goals could be part of a more structured professional development experience such as with graduate nurses in a TTP or for nurses who are on orientation. This briefing could also be integrated into handoff reports or shift change reports. Briefing with goal clarification allows for nurses to ask clarifying questions or begin preparing a plan on how to tackle the clinical day.

Nurse leaders who begin the day with a prebriefing also support nurses becoming more situationally aware of their learning and clinical environment, model how to interact with clients, and can be more in tuned to the unit dynamics to decrease anxiety among the nursing team and increase overall learning opportunities.[7] This step contextualizes the larger clinical environment, fostering a deeper understanding of the patients' conditions and the decisions that need to be made.

2. Establish psychological safety

Creating a safe environment is pivotal for effective learning in the clinical setting,[4,5] and sets the tone for nurses to be allowed to ask questions. Creating this safe environment is important so that nurses can feel comfortable expressing limitations in their own practice without the fear of being ridiculed. Safe environments are especially relevant in the high-pressure hospital setting such as an intensive care unit, where novice nurses may feel overwhelmed. Maintaining the psychological environment will allow for crucial conversations to take place where the novice nurse will be open to feedback.[8] In addition, it will also allow novice nurses to feel more comfortable seeking constructive feedback or asking questions without fear of judgment or reprimand, increasing the likelihood they will seek assistance in high-risk circumstances, and potentially preventing errors or negative outcomes.

Nurse educators and leaders can promote psychological safety in a variety of ways in the clinical or practice settings. For example, by conducting prebriefing they make themselves accessible for nurses. This accessibility promotes opportunity for communication and approachability. They can also use Socratic, open-ended, or probing questions to promote dialogue and assess understanding without being judgmental or demeaning to nurses. When concerns, limitations, or mistakes are brought to the attention of the nurse leaders or educators, they can include the nurses involved in the process to address them to help them learn from the situation instead of fearing punishment. By seeking these learning opportunities, nurses will be more likely to engage in finding ways to improve the outcomes. They will then be more likely to communicate and share difficulties in the future.

3. Familiarize with technology and equipment

If the simulation involves technical equipment, prebriefing provides an opportunity for participants to familiarize themselves with the tools they will use during the scenario. This familiarity reduces confusion during the simulation and allows students to focus on patient care. This concept carries over to the hospital setting. It is important to review unfamiliar equipment with nurses to ensure patient safety. Orienting nurses on infrequently used or new equipment will also assist in building competency of its use and promoting situational awareness. Having the nurses become more situationally aware can lead to increased clinical judgment and competent nursing care.[7]

Benefits for Practicing Nurses

Prebriefing encourages nurses to critically analyze patient care prior to starting their clinical shift. This anticipatory thinking enhances their clinical judgment and decision-making skills, both of which are essential for safe and effective patient care. This analysis also promotes reflective practice which assists in the continuous improvement of their professional practice and growth. For example, nurse educators can incorporate structured conversations on clinical reasoning, ethical dilemmas, and communication strategies in the prebriefing process. This approach enhances not only clinical skills but also reflective practice among novice nurses. It allows novices to expand their confidence and competence in nursing.

A final benefit of adding prebriefing into the clinical environments is increasing the leadership skills of the charge nurse. Effective prebriefing equips the charge nurse with strategies to communicate expectations clearly and promote a collaborative working environment among the nursing staff. Charges nurse can optimize interprofessional team dynamics that can lead to safe patient care and improve clinical competence.

SUMMARY

Implementing the concepts of prebriefing into simulation and nursing practice can promote psychological safety and promote better professional and team development in healthcare environments. While prebriefing has a specific need in simulation conducted in both clinical and academic settings, it also can serve a great purpose in nursing practice. Nurse educators and leaders at all levels can utilize the concepts of developing a prebriefing plan and psychological safety to promote communication and learning with the goal of creating safer clinical environments for patients and staff.

Simulation can be used to assess clinical competencies, transition new nurses to practice, and testing system processes and equipment. Threading simulation best practices concepts through the clinical setting are ideal for developing deeper learning opportunities, developing nurses' leadership and education skills, and creating safe learning and practice environments. Incorporating a standard prebriefing method and plan that carries throughout the clinical environment may be one way to decrease stress and anxiety of the nursing team and promote a psychologically safe working environment.

CLINICS CARE POINTS

- Reflect on your own level of expertise and competency in simulation.
- Assess your learners and their level of knowledge, expertise, and competency. Use this assessment to guide their experience.

- Prepare learners for the simulation experience through orientation, providing logistics and allowing for questions.
- Clarify goals and learning objectives in simulation and in the clinical practice setting.
- Create a safe learning environment by reviewing expectations, providing feedback, and seeking input and new ideas.
- Orient new nurses to any new equipment or technology they will use in simulation and/or the clinical setting.

DISCLOSURE

The authors have no commercial or financial conflicts of interest to report and have not received any funding for this project.

REFERENCES

1. Morse C, Fey M, Kardong-Edgren S, et al. The changing landscape of simulation-based education. Am J Nurs 2019;119(8):42–8.
2. Harper MG, Bodine J, Monachino A. The Effectiveness of Simulation Use in Transition to Practice Nurse Residency Programs: A Review of Literature From 2009 to 2018. J Nurses Pro Dev 2021;37(6):329–40.
3. INACSL Standards Committee. Healthcare Simulation Standards of Best Practice™. Clin Simul Nurs 2021. https://doi.org/10.1016/j.ecns.2021.08.018.
4. McDermott DS, Ludlow J, Horsley E, Meakim C. Healthcare simulation standards of best practiceTM prebriefing: preparation and briefing. Clin Simul Nurs 2021; 58:9–13.
5. Rudolph JW, Raemer DB, Simon R, et al. Establishing a safe container for learning in simulation: the role of the presimulation briefing. Int J Healthc Simul 2014;9(6): 339–49.
6. Edmondson A. Psychological safety and learning behavior in work teams. Adm Sci Q 1999;44(2):350–83.
7. Potter AL, Dreifuerst KT, Woda A. Developing Situation Awareness in Simulation Prebriefing. J Nurs Educ 2022;61(5):250–6.
8. Eller S, Rudolph J, Barwick S, et al. Leading change in practice: how "longitudinal prebriefing" nurtures and sustains in situ simulation programs. Adv Simul 2023; 8(1):1–9.

The Essentials of Debriefing and Reflective Practice

Mary K. Fey, PhD, RN, CHSE-A, ANEF[a],*,
Kate J. Morse, PhD, MSN, RN, CHSE, ACNP-Ret[b]

KEYWORDS

- Debriefing • Clinical debriefing • Reflective learning • In-situ simulation
- Clinical teaching

KEY POINTS

- Learning does not happen in simulation without debriefing.
- A debriefing discussion has 3 main phases.
- In addition to learning in a simulation laboratory, simulation can be done in patient care areas, a technique known as in-situ simulation.
- Debriefing techniques can be used to debrief actual clinical practice as well as simulation.

INTRODUCTION/HISTORY/DEFINITIONS/BACKGROUND

Debriefing is an approach to reflective learning with roots in "After Action Reviews" in the military[1] and in the aviation industry.[2] Health professions educators adopted and have continued to hone debriefing skills as simulation-based education (SBE) became a standard part of educating clinicians. In recent years, the same debriefing practices that are used in simulation are used to debrief actual clinical care. Debriefing is broadly defined as a collaborative process in which actions, thoughts, and emotions are retrospectively examined for the purpose of developing clinical judgment and critical thinking skills.[3] In their seminal article, Fanning and Gaba[4] described debriefing as a guided reflective discussion that attempts to bridge the gap between experiencing an event and making sense of it, encouraging the metacognitive skills that lead to the development of expertise. Early studies demonstrated that debriefing following simulation is essential to learning. In fact, early empirical studies[5–7] demonstrated that learning does not occur in SBE in the absence of debriefing.

The practice of debriefing in SBE builds on years of research on reflective practice more broadly. From this earlier study come the terms "reflection in action" and

[a] Principal Faculty, Center for Medical Simulation, Boston, MA, USA; [b] Experiential Learning and Innovation, College of Nursing & Health Professions, Drexel University, 60 North 36th Street, Philadelphia, PA 19104, USA
* Corresponding author. Center for Medical Simulation, 100 1st Street, Boston, MA 02129.
E-mail address: maryfey777@gmail.com

Nurs Clin N Am 59 (2024) 391–400
https://doi.org/10.1016/j.cnur.2024.01.008
0029-6465/24/© 2024 Elsevier Inc. All rights reserved.

nursing.theclinics.com

"reflection on action."[8] Reflection in action refers to the in-the-moment thought processes that take place as professionals assess their current situation to determine if they are meeting their objective(s). In the context of patient care, clinicians use reflection in action to determine if they are on the right track with treatment and care decisions, for example, Have I given enough fluid to bring up the blood pressure? Am I seeing the verbal and nonverbal cues that tell me the patient understands what I am telling them? Reflection on action occurs after a care episode, as events and actions are reviewed to determine if the correct actions were taken and if the desired outcomes were achieved. Both types of reflection are important to the development of nursing clinical judgment.[9] Debriefing following SBE or a care episode is a form of reflection on action.

The International Nursing Association for Clinical Simulation and Learning has published Simulation Standards of Best Practice, including a Standard for The Debriefing Process. The criteria required to meet the standard include that it is

- Planned as an integral part of the SBE experience
- Facilitated by a person who is competent to do so
- Conducted in a manner that facilitates reflection and analysis
- A method that is based on theoretic frameworks[10]

DISCUSSION
Methods of Debriefing

There are several methods of debriefing in current use in simulation that are based on educational theories. Across these different methods, there are commonalities in the structure: there is an initial intake phase that sets up the reflective discussion to follow; there is an analysis phase in which actions and thought processes are reviewed and discussed; and a summary phase in which take-away lessons and future practice improvements are identified. All methods of debriefing share the goal of understanding the thinking behind the actions that were observed during the simulation. Several of the methods in use are Debriefing with Good Judgment,[11] Promoting Excellence And Reflective Learning in Simulation,[12] and Debriefing for Meaningful Learning.[13]

In debriefings, the initial phase helps the learners transition from the action-oriented simulation case to the reflective learning conversation that is about to take place. During this time, learners are encouraged to express their feelings in response to a facilitator question such as "How are you feeling right now?" This allows the emotional activation that occurred during the simulation to dissipate. It may also be the time to ascertain what the learners found most challenging by asking, "What was difficult for you during that case?" This allows the facilitator to do an in-the-moment learning need assessment before proceeding with the debriefing. This phase is brief (several minutes).

Following the initial phase, the facilitator guides the learners through an analysis of the case. During this analytical phase, the facilitator's primary goal is to understand why the learners took the actions they took by asking open-ended questions. Understanding the thought processes that led to the observable actions allows the educator to "diagnose" the learning need so that they can then "treat" the actual learning need. For example, there are several possible reasons that a clinician might deviate from the expected actions during a simulation. It could be a case of lack of situational awareness, poor communication in the team, and a lack of understanding about the pathophysiology or treatment protocols. If the facilitator assumes a knowledge deficit and proceeds to lecture on the topic when the actual problem was poor communication, then the learning opportunity is missed. Once the learning need has been diagnosed, the facilitator can then lead a discussion focused on solutions that will improve practice in the future. One technique that can be used for questioning that will get to the thought processes of the learner is the advocacy-inquiry questioning technique. After first introducing the topic, the facilitator asks the advocacy-inquiry question by first stating their observation in factual terms, then explaining to the learners why they are concerned with this point, and then inviting the learners to reflect on and share their thinking. See **Table 1** for advocacy-inquiry structure and suggested scripting.

Debriefing and reflective practice

It is important to note that facilitators should not only focus on errors in debriefing. In recent patient safety oriented publications, clinicians are being encouraged to learn from the successes of good clinical practice by studying error-free performance.[14,15] Fey and Johnson[16] provide guidance on debriefing positive performance using the cognitive task analysis approach. In this approach, the facilitator focuses on helping learners reflect on the thought processes that led to a good decision, that is, what assessment data they noted, how they interpreted that data, and how they decided on a course of action. This reinforces good practice. See **Table 2** for a guide to the phases of debriefing.

The final phase is the summary phase in which learners are asked to state their take-home lessons and/or discuss how they will integrate the new learning into their practice. In this phase, the facilitator may say, "Based on the topics we have covered, what are your main take-home points? How will they influence your practice going forward?"

See **Table 3** for a guide to debriefing positive performance.

SETTINGS FOR DEBRIEFING IN SIMULATION-BASED EDUCATION

SBE has been broadly adopted in prelicensure and advanced practice nursing education. Many healthcare agencies have also integrated simulation into the orientation and development of individual clinicians and healthcare teams. With practicing clinicians, simulation and debriefing can take place in simulation centers or in the clinical practice environment in which clinicians practice, which is called in-situ

Table 1 Advocacy-inquiry questioning technique	
Simulation case events: A patient with a pulmonary embolism developed worsening shortness of breath. During the simulation, the team members were focused mainly on the thrombolytic aspect of treatment. The patient's oxygen delivery was set at 4 L/min, and no one increased the oxygen delivery despite falling oxygen saturation readings	
Preview	Letting learners know the topic that is about to be discussed: *"I would like to talk about managing oxygenation"*
Advocacy[1]	A statement with the objective facts: *"I saw that the patient's O_2 saturation was 86% and I did not see anyone increase the oxygen"*
Advocacy[2]	Your concerns about the impact of this action on the patient: *"I was worried that the hypoxia was going to continue to get worse without it"*
Inquiry	An open-ended question to invite them to share their thinking at the time: *"Can you walk me through your thinking at the time?"*

Table 2 Phases of debriefing	
Phase of Debriefing	**Possible Scripting**
Phase 1: Transition from simulation to reflective debriefing	"Thanks for your participation in that simulation case. How are you feeling right now?"
Phase 2: Analysis phase	"As we get started with the analysis of the case, I am curious: what parts of the simulation did you find challenging?" (this is a mini needs assessment) For each topic, begin with an open-ended advocacy/inquiry question (**Table 1** for structure of advocacy-inquiry)
Phase 3: Summary phase	"Based on what we talked about today, what are the take-home points you will incorporate into your practice going forward?"

simulation. Although both places in which simulation takes place share the same objective, that is, to examine practice for the purpose of improvement, their approaches can differ.

Simulation Center-Based Debriefing

SBE that occurs in a simulation center has several advantages versus SBE done in patient care areas.

- Clinicians are scheduled to be in simulation, so the SBE event is less likely to be canceled because of heavy patient loads
- Participants can focus solely on the SBE because they are away from the demands of the patient care area.
- In this setting, the SBE facilitator often has more time for both the simulation and the debriefing, and the learners are less likely to be distracted
- There are no potential safety hazards from mixing up simulated equipment and supplies with "real" patient care items
- There is no risk of patients or family member being inadvertently affected by seeing the simulation
- There is potentially better facilitation of debriefings because of dedicated simulation staff[17]

In-situ Debriefing

In-situ simulations, which take place in the actual patient care area has several advantages over SBE done in a simulation center.

- Staff are already in the patient care area, so there is no time lost in getting to a simulation center
- It enhances team learning for the intact team(s) who practice there
- Latent patient safety threats in the environment can be uncovered and corrected
- Can be less expensive due to the availability of supplies and equipment.

One of the main disadvantages of in-situ simulation is that, because it often occurs during the staff's work hours, it must be much more time efficient. This generally means less time for both the simulation and the debriefing. In this case, the facilitator must limit the number of topics that can be explored during the debriefing.[18] Where a typical center-based simulation and debriefing might take 1 hour (20 minutes for the

Table 3
Debriefing positive performance[16]

Debriefer Dialog	Learner Dialog	Data Gathered from Learner Dialog
Context: In a simulation case, a learner did an outstanding job with an upset family member who had the potential to become very disruptive		
P: "Paul, I would like to talk about your approach with the family member"	"Well, I could see them getting restless in the chair and I heard their voice getting louder and louder, so I knew they were getting more upset. They were not even able to listen to us. This could be a problem.	Cues that the situation was escalating: Restlessness Increasing volume of voice Not responding to requests from team Family member interfering with team
A[1]: "I saw that when the family member did not sit down, you engaged with them in a way that seemed to calm them."	Once they got out of their chair and came to the bedside, the behavior really made it hard for the team to work—the team leader could not pay attention to the situation and the family	Goal: control the chaos by reallocating roles—the remaining 3 team members would be able to handle the IV fluids, VS, and communication with provider
A[2]: "It really helped the team that you were able to stay with the family member so that the team could communicate more clearly."	member at the same time and none of us could hear her anymore. It was just too chaotic now.	
I: "I am curious what was going on in your mind then? Listen...."	I was torn about what to do, because I wanted to stay there and continue manage the IV fluids, since the BP was so low.	
	We all agreed that the most helpful role for me would be to stay with the family."	
"Right, that was very effective. Now, talk to me about your approach with the family member"	"First of all, I know what it is like.... I have been the parent standing next to the stretcher in the ER...it is awful.	Strategies: Find empathetic connection Stay calm and engage: if I am calm, it will calm them; if I go with them, they will step away from the bedside, too
	Well, I knew that shouting at them would only escalate the situation, so I purposely kept my voice and manner quiet and calm, hoping they would mirror that. I made eye contact and led them to the chair, alongside one for me."	Establish a common goal with family member—care of their loved one

(continued on next page)

Table 3
(continued)

Debriefer Dialog	Learner Dialog	Data Gathered from Learner Dialog

Debriefer data analysis and synthesis:
"So, this is what you have just told me:
• The cues that indicate escalating behavior include restlessness, increasing volume of voice, and not responding to requests from team
• The line that cannot be crossed is behavior that interferes with patient care; at that point, it becomes a priority to deescalate the behavior
• Strategies to use include
  ○ Check in with team about changes in roles
  ○ Find an empathetic connection with the family member
  ○ Keep your voice low and calm
  ○ Lead them away and stay with them
  ○ Establish a common goal—ensuring that their loved one gets the best care
  ○ Monitor the situation
Anything else you would like to add?"*		

simulation and 40 minutes for debriefing), in-situ simulations are more commonly shorter (5–10 minutes for the simulation and 15–20 minutes for the debriefing).

There is not a "better" place for simulation. Rather, the choice of place should be based on what the objective of the simulation is.[19]

DEBRIEFING ACTUAL CLINICAL EXPERIENCES

Increasingly, debriefing in the actual clinical environment following episodes of patient care is being recognized as a powerful learning tool. Clinical debriefing (CD) has been shown to positively enhance team functioning and patient outcomes.[20] The type of CD discussed here refers to planned debriefings, not debriefing after a traumatic event. Debriefing following a traumatic event is called "critical incident stress debriefing." Critical incident stress debriefing (CISD) is a facilitator-led group process conducted after a traumatic event, when participants are under stress from exposure to the event.[21] CISD may be done following events such as death of a child from nonaccidental injury or acts of workplace violence.

CDs may be planned for low-volume, high-acuity events such as cardiac arrest and resuscitation, intubations, or for new clinical protocols such as those that were seen in the initial phase of the COVID-19 pandemic. For clinical preceptors who are orienting new staff members, a planned debriefing at the end of each orientation day or at other regular intervals can add the important element of reflective practice in a situation in which there is rapid learning occurring. Because of this rapid learning, the new staff member is likely to have many developmental learning needs. Debriefing can be a way to surface these learning needs, if it is done in a way that supports reflection and allows vulnerability in learning. It is a willingness to be vulnerable that allows a person in a new role to either admit they do not know something or ask for help. In order to do this, the learner must trust that their vulnerability will not be met with shaming or humiliation. In other words, the learner must feel psychologically safe. In fact, when learners do not feel psychologically safe, they are more likely to withdraw and disengage from the learning environment.[22]

There are several key behaviors a clinical preceptor can engage in that will foster a sense of psychological safety. They are as follows:

- Building the relationship and setting up learners for success by providing clear expectations for the work to be done, and the expected level of mastery. For example, when guiding a new acute care nurse practitioner before doing their first independent history and physical the preceptor may say, "I would like you to do this H&P independently. What I am looking for is a thorough social history as well as medical history. When you are doing the physical examination, please be sure to check closely for hepato/splenomegaly. Let us aim for you to get that done in 1 hour. If you think you need to consult with me at any point, I will be right here, just call me in. What questions do you have?"
- Encouraging engagement in learning by modeling humility and encouraging learner autonomy. Humility on the part of the more senior person is a way of acknowledging gaps in knowledge, which normalizes the learning process and models lifelong learning. Autonomy demonstrates that the preceptor trusts them enough to give them an appropriate level of independence, which has been shown to promote feelings of belonging and engagement in learners.
- Reinforcing every effort as a learning opportunity and proving frequent feedback.[22]

When providing feedback, the advocacy-inquiry method can be used. Imagine that the new nurse practitioner referenced above completed the H&P but it took them

45 minutes (not the 30 minutes as requested). An advocacy-inquiry approach to debriefing that may be as follows:

Let us talk about time and efficiency now. The goal was to get the H&P done within 60 minutes. I see that it took closer to 90 minutes. Once your caseload increases, taking that long for an H&P will have you behind schedule all day. Talk to me about how you managed time in there.

A recent consensus discussion was held to define parameters for CD, and recommendations are as follows:

- Formulate criteria for when and when not to debrief. CD, as opposed to CISD, seeks to learn from everyday work practices.
- Clearly articulate the purpose and the value of CD to those who will be involved.
- Emphasize a psychologically safe environment.
- Use a consistent approach to promote familiarity and decrease cognitive load for both facilitators and learners.
- Limit the number of topics, and establish a method to turn learning from debriefing into meaningful organizational/environmental changes.
- Focus on team-based factors and collective problem solving, rather than individual errors.
- Be aware of the legalities of the discussion and subsequent documentation. In some jurisdictions, these types of discussion may be discoverable; CD programs must be aware of local legal requirements.[20]

SUMMARY

Debriefing is a powerful tool that builds metacognitive skills to create the reflective practitioner needed in today's complex, fast-paced healthcare system. Although usually associated with simulation, debriefing techniques can and should also be used to examine and improve actual clinical care.

CLINICS CARE POINTS

- Debriefing is driven by curiosity—keep an open mind and ask open-ended questions
- Debriefing should be transparent—do not expect learners/clinicians to "guess what you are thinking"
- Consider all perspectives when exploring issues
- Debriefing is not about "telling them what they did wrong"—it is about exploring the many contextual issues that interfere with care delivery
- Remember to debrief good performance as well as errors

DISCLOSURE

Dr K.J. Morse has no commercial or financial conflicts of interest to report. There are no funding sources to report. Dr M.K. Fey has no commercial or financial conflicts of interest to report. There are no funding sources to report.

REFERENCES

1. Darling M, Parry C, Moore J. Learning in the thick of it. Harv Bus Rev 2005; 83(7):84.

2. Dismukes RK, Smith GM. Facilitation and debriefing in aviation training and operations. Philadelphia, PA: Routledge; 2017.
3. Lopreiato J. Healthcare simulation dictionary, Society for Simulation in Healthcare 2018. Available at: ssih.org/dictionary. Accessed April 22, 2018.
4. Fanning RM, Gaba DM. The role of debriefing in simulation-based learning. Simulat Healthc J Soc Med Simulat 2007;2(2):115–25.
5. Mahmood T, Darzi A. The learning curve for a colonoscopy simulator in the absence of any feedback: no feedback, no learning. Surgical Endoscopy And Other Interventional Techniques 2004;18:1224–30.
6. Savoldelli GL, Naik VN, Park J, et al. Value of debriefing during simulated crisis management: oral versusvideo-assisted oral feedback. The Journal of the American Society of Anesthesiologists 2006;105(2):279–85.
7. Shinnick MA, Woo M, Horwich TB, et al. Debriefing: The most important component in simulation? Clinical simulation in Nursing 2011; 7(3):e105–11.
8. Schön DA. The reflective practitioner: how professionals think in action. Philadelphia, PA: Routledge; 2017.
9. Tanner CA. Thinking like a nurse: A research-based model of clinical judgment in nursing. J Nurs Educ 2006;45(6):204–11.
10. INACSL Standards Committee, Healthcare Simulation Standards of Best Practice: The Debriefing Process. 2021. 58: p. 27-32. Available at: https://www.inacsl.org/healthcare-simulation-standards. Accessed April 22, 2023.
11. Rudolph JW, Simon R, Dufresne RL, et al. There's no such thing as "nonjudgmental" debriefing: a theory and method for debriefing with good judgment. Simulat Healthc J Soc Med Simulat 2006;1(1):49–55.
12. Eppich W, Cheng A. Promoting Excellence and Reflective Learning in Simulation (PEARLS): development and rationale for a blended approach to health care simulation debriefing. Simulat Healthc J Soc Med Simulat 2015;10(2): 106–15.
13. Dreifuerst KT. Using debriefing for meaningful learning to foster development of clinical reasoning in simulation. J Nurs Educ 2012;51(6):326–33.
14. Hollnagel E, Wears RL, Braithwaite J. From Safety-I to Safety-II: a white paper. The resilient health care net: published simultaneously by the University of Southern Denmark. Australia: University of Florida, USA, and Macquarie University; 2015.
15. Dieckmann P, Patterson M, Lahlou S, et al. Variation and Adaptation: Learning from Success in patient-safety oriented simulation training. Advances in Simulation 2017;2(21):1–14.
16. Fey M, Johnson BK. They didn't do anything wrong! What will I talk about? International Journal of Healthcare Simulation 2023;1–6 (null).
17. Dieckmann P, Sharara-Chami R, Ersdal HL. Debriefing practices in simulation-based education. Clinical Education for the Health Professions: Theory and Practice 2020;1–17.
18. Sørensen JL, Østergaard D, LeBlanc V, et al. Design of simulation-based medical education and advantages and disadvantages of in situ simulation versus off-site simulation. BMC Med Educ 2017;17:1–9.
19. Brazil V. Translational simulation: not 'where?'but 'why?'A functional view of in situ simulation. Advances in Simulation 2017;2(1):1–5.
20. Coggins A, Zaklama R, Szabo RA, et al. Twelve tips for facilitating and implementing clinical debriefing programmes. Med Teach 2021;43(5): 509–17.

21. Occupational Safety and Health Administration. Critical Incident Stress Guide. Available at: https://www.osha.gov/emergency-preparedness/guides/critical-incident-stress#:~:text=Critical%20Incident%20Stress%20Debriefing%20(CISD, under%20stress%20from%20trauma%20exposure).
22. McClintock AH, Fainstad TL, Jauregui J. Clinician teacher as leader: creating psychological safety in the clinical learning environment for medical students. Acad Med 2022;97(11S):S46–53.

Implementing Simple and Effective Simulation Experiences

Darla Gruben, EdD(c), MSN, CHSE, CNE*,[1],
Elizabeth Wells-Beede, PhD, RN, C-EFM, CHSE-A, CNE, ACUE, FAAN[1]

KEYWORDS

- Bedside simulation • Hospital simulation • In situ simulation • Healthcare simulation
- Nursing education

KEY POINTS

- Considerations and utilization of The Healthcare Simulation Standards of Best Practice.
- Overcoming barriers for the bedside nurse and educator.
- Practicing nurses can utilize in situ bedside simulations for interdisciplinary training with high-risk, low-volume cases.
- Simulation at the bedside to demonstrate improved patient outcomes with evidence-based practice to inform the research.

INTRODUCTION

Implementing simple and effective nursing simulation experiences at the bedside or in a simulation training center in a hospital setting can be an impactful way to enhance skill development, encourage critical thinking, and improve patient safety. Historically, high-fidelity simulations have been employed in the hospital setting for orientation programs, continuing education, staff development, nursing professional development, high-risk, low-volume scenarios, and team building.[1] According to Kelsey and Claus,[2] bedside simulations allow practicing nurses to refine tasks, increase confidence in skills, build teamwork, and identify process gaps. Klenke-Borgmann and colleagues[3] found in their pilot study that nurse residents experienced increased confidence in their prioritization, time management, and delegation abilities after virtual simulation and then could directly apply this knowledge to their practice at the bedside. In situ simulations can positively impact nurses' confidence, improve nursing practice in recognizing signs

College of Nursing, The University of North Texas Health Science Center, Fort Worth, Texas, USA
[1] Present address: 3500 Camp Bowie Boulevard, Fort Worth, TX 76107.
* Corresponding author.
E-mail address: Darla.gruben@unthsc.edu

and symptoms of a deteriorating patient, and initiate interventions to improve patient outcomes.[4] Although the literature is filled with positive rationale for utilizing simulation in the hospital setting, there are often barriers to the bedside practicing nurse participating in simulation. These barriers and solutions will be explored. Applying the Healthcare Simulation Standards of Best Practice (HSSOBP™)[5] will give the bedside practicing nurse, the hospital clinical educator, and the simulation facilitator consistency in implementing and planning effective simulations in the hospital setting.

DEFINITIONS

The following definitions describe 2 simulation settings in a hospital environment.

In Situ Simulation

Simulations taught within the confines of the hospital setting are defined as in situ. In situ simulations are described as simulation-based experiences (SBEs) in the actual clinical environment rather than in a simulation training center to improve patient care.[6,7] In situ simulation education experiences are designed for professional skills development, to enhance teamwork, and to improve patient outcomes where the participants are employed.[7] Implementing the in situ simulation in the exact location where the nurse or team works and patient care occurs increases the fidelity of the simulation.[8] In situ simulations are also implemented to test new equipment, hospital processes, and facility designs to improve patient safety and quality.[9] In situ simulation in the hospital-based setting supports adult learning as an evidence-based method in a safe environment.[4] In situ simulations are sometimes impossible with nursing staffing shortages and an increased census, as there may not be a hospital room to conduct the simulation.

Skills and Simulation Laboratory/Training Center

Hospital settings can also have simulation laboratories or training centers where deliberate practice can hone skills and mastery assessments for the practicing nurse to determine the competence of knowledge, skills, and attitudes of professional practice. Simulation laboratories become critical when hospital beds are at capacity, and space is still needed to practice using new equipment or procedures in the hospital. Having participants in their employment settings can make the experience more meaningful to the participants using their equipment, rooms, and teams. Participants in a hospital setting are people on a healthcare team who work together with the intention of improving patient care outcomes. Participants include nurses, providers, clinical nurse assistants, respiratory therapists, unit clerks, physical therapists, occupational therapists, pharmacists, and administrators. Determining who the participants will be depends on the objectives and the purpose of the simulation, which will be explored more in depth in later discussion.

SIMULATION OPPORTUNITIES IN THE HOSPITAL SETTING

There are many opportunities and ideas for simulation at the bedside, in the simulation laboratory/training centers, and in situ. Simulations are also used in response to sentinel events and medication errors to practice correct processes and procedures to improve patient outcomes in the future. Current morbidity/mortality rates can also determine the need for simulations. These unfortunate experiences can evolve into simulation scenarios by creating case studies based on root cause analysis. The end goal of all simulations is to improve patient outcomes. The following (**Box 1**) is a list of simulation ideas easily implemented in the hospital setting that

---

Box 1
Simulation ideas easily implemented in the hospital setting

- General Hospital Orientation
- National Patient Safety Goals (Joint Commission)
- New Graduate Residency Programs
- Continuing education for staff nurse development
- Ancillary support staff development
- Train the trainer professional development
- High-risk low-volume simulations
- Team building
- Interprofessional development
- Deliberate practice of skills
- Mastery and competency checks
- Practice with new equipment
- New hospital process practice
- Systems thinking activity (Turn tabletop activities into a live event)
- Sentinel new hospital process practice
- Medication errors prevention with near miss events
- Risk reduction and patient safety initiatives
- Therapeutic communication
- TeamSTEPPS
- Miscommunication errors (situation background assessment repeat [SBAR]-shift report practice)
- After action reports
- Difficult conversations
- Ethical considerations
- Civility and workplace violence solutions

---

are guided by the HSSOBP™ Facilitation and HSSOBP™ Operations to help ensure competent facilitators and technicians trained in simulation.

CHALLENGES AND BARRIERS TO IMPLEMENTING SIMULATION

Many goals and possibilities exist for using simulation in the hospital setting. There are also barriers to conducting simulations for the bedside nurse, whether in situ or a skills and simulation laboratory/training center setting. The following (**Table 1**) lists problems and solutions to consider when implementing bedside simulation.

STANDARDS, MODELS, TEMPLATES, THEORIES, INSTRUMENTS, AND FRAMEWORKS FOR SIMULATION

Simulation can be expensive even if considered simple; therefore, seeking grants for funding simulation programs is often essential. Using best practices will support,

Table 1
Problems and solutions for simulation

Problems	Solutions
The unit census is unpredictable; therefore, it can be challenging to conduct in situ simulations, especially if the unit does not have an empty bed to conduct the simulation[4,9]	An alternative plan is to conduct the SBE in a breakroom or conference room. In situ simulation training utilizing familiar surroundings enhanced the participants' knowledge, skills, abilities, and confidence[4] Using a patient room where the participants work reinforced habits such as hand hygiene[4]
Practicing nurses providing direct care may have difficulty leaving the unit to attend a simulation[9]	Virtual simulation or screen-based simulation could be a solution for nursing residency training.[3] Virtual simulations do not take staff away from the unit; however, consideration for compensation for their time must be addressed by administrators Rochlen and colleagues recommended extended reality-based simulation training for critical events (high acuity, low-frequency events) that are difficult to create in real life[12]
Nurses may not get compensated to attend a training session if the session is not on a day they are already scheduled[9]	Use hospital survey data to garner administrative support and seek grant funding for additional training[13]
Simulation training for staff is a considerable commitment in time, energy, and resources	Ensure as much as possible that when an event is scheduled, it is not canceled, as these events in the hospital are complex to reschedule
Transporting equipment (manikins and high-fidelity simulators) can also be a challenge utilizing in situ simulation[14]	Ensuring technical support is also a consideration to overcome this barrier[4] The HSSOBP™ Operations[11] discusses sustainability, people, and processes necessary to implement SBEs
The hospital setting may have minimal resources for simulation technician training, the facilitators' and educators' professional development support, and the hiring of standardized patients (SPs)	Partnering with volunteer organizations, community college theater departments, high-school fine arts departments, and community thespians are a solution to recruiting and training SPs. Academic collaborations with universities and colleges to assist with grant funding can support hospital simulation programs and foster partnerships to improve patient outcomes and train the healthcare team

inform, and foster the scholarship of simulation. To implement simple and effective simulations, the practicing nurse, clinical educator, and simulation facilitator can employ HSSOBP™ (**Table 2**), Models, templates, theories, instruments, and frameworks for simulation planning (**Table 3**) can also be utilized for simulation. These rich resources cited in **Tables 2** and **3** are based on evidence to support participants' psychological safety, achieve improved patient outcomes, and inform the literature with simulation research.

Table 2
Healthcare simulation standards of best practice

Standards	Website or Reference
HSSOBP™ Operations[11]	INACSL Standards Committee, Charnetski M, Jarvill M. Healthcare simulation standards of best practice™ operations. *Clin Sim in Nurs* 2021;58:33–39. Available at https://doi.org/10.1016/j.ecns.2021.08.012. Accessed November 23, 2023.
HSSOBP™ Outcomes and Objectives[15]	NACSL Standards Committee, Miller C, Deckers C, Jones M, Wells-Beede E, McGee E. Healthcare simulation standards of best practice™ outcomes and objectives. *Clin Sim in Nurs* 2021;58:40–44. Available at https://doi.org/10.1016/j.ecns.2021.08.013. Accessed November 23, 2023.
HSSOBP™ Simulation Design[16]	INACSL Standards Committee, Watts PI, McDermott, DS, Alinier G, Charnetski M, Ludlow J, Horsley E, Meakim C, Nawathe P. Healthcare simulation standards of best practice™ simulation design. Clin Sim in Nurs 2021;58:14–21. Available at https://doi.org/10.1016/j.ecns.2021.08.009. Accessed November 23, 2023.
HSSOBP™ Prebriefing: Preparation and Briefing[17]	INACSL Standards Committee, McDermott D, Ludlow J, Horsley E, Meakim C. Healthcare simulation standards of best practice™ prebriefing: Preparation and briefing. *Clin Sim in Nurs* 2021;58:9–13. Available at https://doi.org/10.1016/j.ecns.2021.08.008. Accessed November 23, 2023.
HSSOBP™ Facilitation[10]	INACSL Standards Committee, Persico L, Belle A, DiGregorio H, Wilson-Keates B, Shelton C. Healthcare simulation standards of best practice™ facilitation. Clin Sim in Nurs 2021;58:22–26 Available at https://doi.org/10.1016/j.ecns.2021.08.010. Accessed November 23, 2023.
HSSOBP™ The Debriefing Process[18]	INACSL Standards Committee, Decker S, Alinier G, Crawford SB, Gordon RM, Jenkins D, Wilson C. Healthcare simulation standards of best practice™ the debriefing process. *Clin Sim in Nur* 2021;58:27–32 Available at https://doi.org/10.1016/j.ecns.2021.08.011. Accessed November 23, 2023.
HSSOBP™ Evaluation of Learning and Performance[19]	INACSL Standards Committee, McMahon E, Jimenez FA, Lawrence K, Victor J. Healthcare simulation standards of best practice™ evaluation of learning and performance. *Clin Sim in Nur* 2021;58:54–56 Available at https://doi.org/10.1016/j.ecns.2021.08.016. Accessed November 23, 2023.
HSSOBP™ Professional Development[20]	INACSL Standards Committee, Hallmark B, Brown M, Peterson D, Fey M, Decker S, Wells-Beede E, Britt T, Hardie L, Shum C, Arantes H, Charnetski, M, Morse C.

(continued on next page)

Table 2 (*continued*)	
Standards	**Website or Reference**
	Healthcare simulation standards of best practice™ professional development. Clin Sim in Nur 2021;58:5–8. Available at: https://doi.org/10.1016/j.ecns.2021.08.007. Accessed November 23, 2023.
Healthcare Simulation Standards Endorsement	https://www.inacsl.org/healthcare-simulation-standards-endorsement

STEP-BY-STEP CONSIDERATIONS
Planning

According to the HSSOBP™ Outcomes and Objectives,[15] an SBE emerges after identifying a need. The learning objectives for the SBE are created from the needs assessment. The needs assessment and the creation of learning objectives and outcomes are essential to develop scenarios needed to achieve the outcomes of the SBE. Simulation planning is required to ensure a successful launch and completion of the simulation-based learning experience. The following steps are defined in the HSSOBP™,[15] and general criteria are included for implementing new simulation opportunities for the hospital setting.

1. Needs assessment: Conduct an initial assessment to determine the specific learning needs, skills to be improved, and the simulation objectives. Needs assessments are critical to creating reliable and valid scenarios. For example, what errors have occurred with the hospital over the last year? What areas have been identified by patient surveys or employee surveys? How do national/regional/state mortality and morbidity rates inform the needs? Has there been a sentinel event?
2. Secure buy-in: Discuss the plan with stakeholders such as nursing staff, hospital administration, and educators to secure their support. This step is covered in the HSSOBP™ Operations.[11] A clear plan for budgeting, sustainability, and resource management will be considered at this step. Knowledge of budgetary constraints and available funds will ensure fiduciary responsibility and facilitate the following 2 steps.
3. Determine the modality and the fidelity of the simulation (**Table 4**).
4. Resource allocation: Identify and allocate resources needed for the simulation. Resources can include manikins, task trainers, virtual reality (VR) headsets, medical equipment, facilitators, and IT support.
5. Determine the resources and equipment needed for SBEs based on the intervention for implementation. The following are just a few types of simulations, each with the required resources for implementation (**Table 4**).

Simulation Design

The HSSOBP™ Simulation Design[16] guides what should occur when designing the simulation. In the hospital setting, the interprofessional team can highlight events that have led to sentinel events. Although catastrophic, these events provide the opportunity for learning and decreasing future errors due to the re-enactment of the event in simulation in the exact setting. The following steps will help guide the process and successful implementation of such scenarios. Simulation might be necessary based on concerns after a root cause analysis, process gaps, or organizational issues

Table 3
Models, templates, theories, instruments, and frameworks for simulation

Models, Templates, Theories, Instruments, and Frameworks	Website or Reference
Society for Simulation in Healthcare Accreditation of Healthcare Simulation Programs	https://www.ssih.org/Credentialing/Accreditation
Considerations for In Situ Simulation (CISS) Framework[7]	Martin A, Cross S, Attoe C. The Use of in situ Simulation in Healthcare Education: Current Perspectives. *Adv Med Educ Pract.* 2020;11:893–903. Published 2020 Nov 27. https://doi.org/10.2147/AMEP.S188258
Critical Conversations: The National League for Nursing Guide for Teaching Thinking[21]	Gross Forneris S and Fey MK. Critical Conversations: The NLN Guide for Teaching Thinking. *Nursing education perspectives.* 2016; 37(5): 248–249. https://doi.org/10.1097/01.NEP.0000000000000069
NLN Jeffries Simulation Theory[22]	Jeffries PR, Rodgers B, Adamson K. NLN Jeffries Simulation Theory: Brief Narrative Description. *Nurs Educ Perspect.* 2015;36(5):292–293. https://doi.org/10.5480/1536-5026-36.5.292
Healthcare Simulation Prebriefing Checkoff Sheet Template	https://www.healthysimulation.com/wp-content/uploads/2019/03/HealthySimulation.com-Prebriefing-Orientation-Checklist.pdf
Repository of Instruments Used in Simulation Research	https://www.inacsl.org/index.php?option=com_content&view=article&id=108:repository-of-instruments&catid=20:site-content&Itemid=149
NLN Simulation Design Template-Revised February 2023	https://www.nln.org/education/education/sirc/sirc/sirc-resources/sirc-tools-and-tips#simtemplate
Healthcare Simulationist Code of Ethics (COE)[23]	Park CS, Murphy, TF, the Code of Ethics Working Group. Healthcare Simulationist Code of Ethics. 2018. Available at https://www.ssih.org/SSH-Resources/Code-of-Ethics Accessed November 22, 2023.
TeamSTEPPS	https://www.ahrq.gov/topics/teamstepps.html
National Patient Safety Goals (Joint Commission)	https://www.jointcommission.org/standards/national-patient-safety-goals/
Interprofessional Education Collaborative	https://www.ipecollaborative.org/ipec-core-competencies

identified in a strengths, weaknesses, opportunities, and threats analysis.[16] The hospital's mission and vision should be considered when designing simulations. What are the goals of the facility? What initiatives need to be highlighted? Are there National Patient and Safety Initiatives for Joint Commission visits that need to be explored? This

Table 4
Types of modalities and fidelity for hospital simulations

Modality	Examples	Best Use in Hospital Setting	Types of Scenarios	Quality Improvement or Patient Safety Drivers.
High fidelity	Gaumard Noelle https://www.gaumard.com/products/obstetrics/noelle	Laboratory setting, possible in situ	Precipitous delivery, shoulder dystocia, and postpartum hemorrhage	Maternal morbidity/mortality rates, Joint Commission, state initiatives, and sentinel events
Midlevel fidelity	Resuscitation Quality Improvement (RQI) system	On units	Codes, Advanced Cardiac Life Support (ACLS), and Basic Life Support (BLS) training	Joint Commission
Low-fidelity	Laerdal Resusci Annie Quality Cardiopulmonary Resuscitation (QCPR) https://laerdal.com/us/products/simulation-training/resuscitation-training/resusci-anne-qcpr/	In situ on units and areas within the hospital such as radiation, operating room (OR), Post Anesthesia Care Unit (PACU) setting	Falls, codes in remote locations, and postpartum hemorrhage	American Heart Association
Task trainers	Injection pad, urinary catheter models (CAE, Limbs and Things) https://www.caehealthcare.com/ https://limbsandthings.com/us	Laboratory areas for skills training and skills fairs, residency programs to up-skill, or new skill training	In conjunction with the above mentioned, if a need exists to give injections, foley insertion, and fundal massage	Core Measures Centers for Disease Control (CDC) Healthcare-Associated Infections (HAIs)
VR	VR Headsets https://www.meta.com/ https://www.apple.com/apple-vision-pro/	On units, in a laboratory setting	Scenarios range from sepsis awareness, OR settings, multipatient, and postpartum hemorrhage. In some hospital settings, collaboration with universities can allow for building personal content	Maternal morbidity/mortality rates, Joint Commission, state initiatives, and sentinel events Core measures CDC HAIs

Screen-based simulation	Sentinel U https://www.sentinelu.com/	Computer laboratories, on unit, laboratory setting	Scenarios are prebuilt and planned with an educational consultant from the vendor	Maternal Morbidity/mortality rates, Joint Commission, state initiatives, and sentinel events Core measures CDC HAIs
Distance simulation	Zoom https://zoom.us/ Microsoft Teams https://www.microsoft.com/en-us/microsoft-teams/group-chat-software	Telehealth Training	Admissions/Discharge Teaching	https://www.ncbi.nlm.nih.gov/pmc/articles/PMC9543712/Health Insurance Portability and Accountability Act HIPAA compliance
Standardized patient	Paid actor/volunteer	Laboratory setting, in situ, on unit preplanned	Scenarios that need assessment on communication or implicit bias	All the above

simulation design standard[16] envelops components of all the HSSOBP™ mentioned thus far in this article. The following steps consider the HSSOBP™ for simulation design[16] with the hospital setting as the lens.

1. Scenario planning based on the needs assessment and the content expertise of the facilitators: Create realistic bedside scenarios that nurses commonly encounter, such as patient deterioration, medication administration, or communication with patients and families. See **Box 1** for a list of simulation opportunities in the hospital setting.
2. Objective setting: Clearly define the objectives to achieve through the simulation. Goals can range from skill improvement, decision-making, and teamwork to communication. Objective setting is critical to scaffold to the next step.
3. Checklists and evaluation rubrics: Develop evaluation tools such as checklists or rubrics for assessing performance and achieving learning outcomes.
4. Prebriefing material: Prepare prebriefing material for participants to prepare them for what to expect, covering the objectives and general flow of the simulation. The pre-brief aims to create a design for the participant to be successful. The objectives should be clear and achievable. For more information on prebriefing, see the Health-care Simulation Standards of Best Practice Prebriefing: Preparation and Briefing.[17]
5. Trial run: Conduct a pilot test with a small group to identify any logistical or technical issues. A complete pilot might not always be possible in the hospital; however, at minimum, systems check or dry one to consider the environment as a psychologically safe space for learning should be considered. This step will help the facilitator or the educator work out the kinks.

Implementation

HSSOBP™ Facilitation[10] explains the criterion emphasizing the importance of having a trained, competent facilitator and an expert in simulation. Kardong-Edgren and Wells-Beede[24] have implored faculty and simulationists that simulation is harmful and unethical to the participants if the facilitator is not competent in simulation. The 6 aspirational values described in the COE are integrity, transparency, mutual respect, professionalism, accountability, and results orientation.[23] The integrity values in the COE state that the simulationist shall work to "eliminate harm to humans, animals, and the environment" (p. 6).[23]

The facilitator will coach and guide the participants. The facilitator will also most often be the one who will utilize the resources in **Table 3** to determine what facilitation methods are needed based on theory and research. The following steps will highlight what has yet to be covered thus far in implementing a simple and effective simulation for the practicing nurse at the bedside.

1. Ensure the facilitator has competency in simulation pedagogy.
2. Assess the needs of the participants: Begin with an orientation session to familiarize participants with the simulation environment, equipment, and objectives.
3. Acknowledge that the SBE is a safe learning environment and mistakes are likely to happen and will be discussed in the debrief.
4. Execute the simulation as planned. Again, make sure to have experienced facilitators to guide the simulation. Assist the participants in achieving learning outcomes.
5. Real-time feedback: Have facilitators and coaches provide real-time feedback during the simulation to guide participants to success.

Debriefing

Debriefing an SBE is necessary to help the learner reflect on the events and, in turn, translate the event to practice, helping to improve practice. Review the HSSOBP™

The Debriefing Process[18] to select a debriefing theory to adopt for the SBE. This debriefing moment is often disregarded, and insufficient time is allowed to help all team members describe their experiences. Some theoretic frameworks in debriefing may not be best suited for in situ. However, it is still vital that whichever debriefing style is considered, the facilitator conducting the debriefing is educated on the framework and allows the learner to reflect. The following are the steps to review for the debriefing steps[18] of implementing simple and effective simulations in the hospital.

1. Plan and structure the debriefing process: Participants should be informed of the debriefing process during the prebrief so they will know what to expect.
2. Immediate feedback: Immediately after the simulation, engage participants in a debriefing session to discuss performance, what went well, what did not, and why. Utilize a debriefing method.
3. Self-assessment and self-reflection: Encourage participants to assess their performance and identify learning points.
4. Review of objectives: Go through the objectives to discuss if participants met the goals and how the facilitators can improve or edit the objectives for future simulations.

Evaluation

HSSOBP™ Evaluation of Learning and Performance[19] guides the facilitator in determining if the participant met the SBE outcomes. Evaluations can be formative or summative in the hospital setting, just like in the academic setting. Deliberate practice or mastery of competency of any of the ideas mentioned in earlier discussion for simulation with different modalities and fidelities will direct the decision-making for the SBE evaluation. The following HSSOBP™[19] will conclude the step-by-step processes for implementing simple and effective simulations in the hospital setting.

1. All facilitators and coaches must be trained in simulation pedagogy, including debriefing and evaluation of simulation, to provide a psychologically safe environment for the SBE.
2. Collect data: Use valid and reliable designed checklists, tools, or rubrics to evaluate each participant's performance. Discussion of a shared mental model for the SBE is also critical for the evaluators to be fair and just to all participants.
3. Participant feedback: Get feedback from participants on the effectiveness of the simulation and areas for improvement. Prepare a survey via electronic resources for the participants to have easy access to complete the feedback before returning to their units to work.
4. Outcome evaluation: Assess whether the participants achieved the learning objectives and how the simulation could impact patient care outcomes.
5. Based on evaluations and feedback, make necessary adjustments to the scenarios, objectives, or execution of the simulation for future SBEs.
6. Document all findings for preparation for article publication, Joint Commission data collection, grant funding requirements, and evidence for continuing education.
7. Yearly or biannually systematic review of simulations to ensure best practices.

Summary

The rationale for simulation in the hospital to improve patient outcomes has been repeatedly demonstrated in the literature. Implementing simple and effective simulation in a hospital setting has many considerations. The checklist for planning a simulation highlights examples (**Table 5**) of the essential components of simulation implementation that can be utilized by the hospital educator or facilitator when

Table 5
Example of checklist for planning a simulation

Action to Perform	Complete	Incomplete
Review and implement HSSOBP™		
Review CISS framework if in situ simulation		
Needs assessment		
Objectives and outcomes		
Determine the type of simulation		
Rubric for measuring outcomes		
Simulation design template		
Proposal for buy-in and budget		
Schedule space		
Invite participants		
Secure equipment		
Prebrief lesson plan from template		
Adopt a debriefing method		
Train all facilitators		
Survey of SBE to participants		
Evaluation of the simulation		
Document all findings of the event		

planning an SBE. This example is based on the HSSOBP™ and the steps discussed in this article.

CLINICS CARE POINTS

- Follow the HSSOBP™[5] to create a psychologically safe environment for the participants and ensure the simulation's goal of improving patient outcomes is achieved.

- By taking a well-planned and structured approach, bedside practicing nurses and educators can implement a simple yet effective nursing simulation experience at the bedside, in line with best practices, educational theory, and research.

- Ensure all activities, results, and modifications are well documented for future reference and for making evidence-based improvements to the simulation program.

DISCLOSURES

The authors have nothing to disclose.

REFERENCES

1. Hallenbeck VJ. Use of high-fidelity simulation for staff education/development: a systematic review of the literature. J Nurses Staff Dev 2012;28(6). 260-E10.
2. Kelsey NC, Claus S. Embedded, in situ simulation improves ability to rescue. Clin Sim in Nurs 2016;12(11):522–7.
3. Klenke-Borgmann L, Setter R, Stubenrauch C, et al. Effect of virtual simulation on nurse residents' prioritization and delegation skills: A pilot study. [published online ahead of print, 2023 Sep 6]. J Nurses Prof Dev 2023. https://doi.org/10.1097/NND.0000000000000985.

4. Lee C, Mowry JL, Maycock SE, et al. The impact of hospital-based in situ simulation on nurses' recognition and intervention of patient deterioration. J Nurses Prof Dev 2019;35(1):18–24.
5. The Healthcare Simulation Standards of Best Practice™ (HSSOBP™). Available In: Education: International Nursing Association for Clinical Simulation (INACSL). 2021. Available at: https://www.inacsl.org/healthcare-simulation-standards-ql. [Accessed 23 November 2023].
6. Kaplan B, Murihead L, Zhang W. Leveraging partnerships: Nursing student veteran-centered simulation in situ. Clin Sim in Nur 2017;13(6):258–63.
7. Martin A, Cross S, Attoe C. The Use of in situ simulation in healthcare education: Current perspectives. Adv Med Educ Pract 2020;11:893–903.
8. Maxworthy JC, Epps C, Okuda Y, et al. Defining excellence in simulation programs. 2. the Netherlands: Wolters Kluwer and SSH Society for Simulation in Healthcare; 2022.
9. Rutherford-Hemming T, Alfes CM. The use of hospital-based simulation in nursing education—A systematic review. Clin Sim in Nurs 2017;13(2):78–89.
10. Persico L, Belle A, DiGregorio H, et al, INACSL Standards Committee. Healthcare simulation standards of best practice™ facilitation. Available at: Clin Sim in Nurs 2021;58:22–6. https://doi.org/10.1016/j.ecns.2021.08.010 . [Accessed 23 November 2023].
11. Charnetski M, Jarvill M, INACSL Standards Committee. Healthcare simulation standards of best practice™ operations. Available at: Clin Sim in Nurs 2021; 58:33–9. https://doi.org/10.1016/j.ecns.2021.08.012 . [Accessed 23 November 2023].
12. Rochlen LR, Putnam EM, Tait AR, et al. Sequential behavioral analysis: A novel approach to help understand clinical decision-making patterns in extended reality simulated scenarios. Simul Healthc 2023;18(5):321–5. https://doi.org/10.1097/SIH.0000000000000686.
13. Connolly AK. Using simulation to hardwire bedside shift report. J Nurs Adm 2017; 47(12):599–601. https://doi.org/10.1097/NNA.0000000000000552.
14. Patterson MD, Blike GT, Nadkarni VM. In situ simulation: Challenges and results. In: Henriksen K, Battles JB, Keyes MA, et al, editors. Advances in patient safety: new directions and alternative approaches. Performance and tools), 3. Rockville, MD: US Agency for Healthcare Research and Quality; 2008.
15. Miller C, Deckers C, Jones M, et al, INACSL Standards Committee. Healthcare simulation standards of best practice™ outcomes and objectives. Available at: Clin Sim in Nurs 2021;58:40–4. https://doi.org/10.1016/j.ecns.2021.08.013 . [Accessed 23 November 2023].
16. Watts PI, McDermott DS, Alinier G, et al, INACSL Standards Committee. Healthcare simulation standards of best practice™ simulation design. Available at: Clin Sim in Nurs 2021;58:14–21. https://doi.org/10.1016/j.ecns.2021.08.009 . [Accessed 23 November 2023].
17. McDermott D, Ludlow J, Horsley E, et al, INACSL Standards Committee. Healthcare simulation standards of best practice™ prebriefing: Preparation and briefing. Available at: Clin Sim in Nurs 2021;58:9–13. https://doi.org/10.1016/j.ecns.2021.08.008 . [Accessed 23 November 2023].
18. Decker S, Alinier G, Crawford SB, et al, INACSL Standards Committee. Healthcare simulation standards of best practice™ the debriefing process. Available at: Clin Sim in Nur 2021;58:27–32. https://doi.org/10.1016/j.ecns.2021.08.011 . [Accessed 23 November 2023].

19. McMahon E, Jimenez FA, Lawrence K, et al, INACSL Standards Committee. Healthcare simulation standards of best practice™ evaluation of learning and performance. Available at: Clin Sim in Nur 2021;58:54–6. https://doi.org/10.1016/j.ecns.2021.08.016 . [Accessed 23 November 2023].

20. Hallmark B, Brown M, Peterson D, et al, INACSL Standards Committee. Healthcare simulation standards of best practice™ professional development. Clin Sim in Nur 2021;58:5–8.

21. Gross Forneris S, Fey MK. Critical Conversations: The NLN Guide for Teaching Thinking. Nurs Educ Perspect 2016;37(5):248–9.

22. Jeffries PR, Rodgers B, Adamson K. NLN Jeffries Simulation Theory: Brief Narrative Description. Nurs Educ Perspect 2015;36(5):292–3.

23. Park CS, Murphy TF. The Code of Ethics Working Group. Healthcare Simulationist Code of Ethics. 2018. Available at: https://www.ssih.org/SSH-Resources/Code-of-Ethics. [Accessed 22 November 2023].

24. Kardong-Edgren S, Wells-Beede E. Stop prelicensure student abuse in simulation. In: Simzine. 2023. Available at: https://simzine.news/focus-en/sim-nurse-en/stop-prelicensure-student-abuse-in-simulation/. [Accessed 23 November 2023].

Designing Evidence-based Simulation Scenarios for Clinical Practice

Carrie Westmoreland Miller, PhD, RN, CNE, CHSE, IBCLC[a,*],
Yuting Lin, PhD, MSN, RN[b], Mary Schafer, MSN, RN, CHSE[c]

KEYWORDS

- Simulation • Design • Pedagogy • Scenario

KEY POINTS

- Simulation design is the framework for quality simulation-based learning experiences.
- Design strategies include needs assessments, consultation with simulation and content experts, and pilot testing before implementation.
- The use of best practices in simulation design is essential to rich learning experiences for learners and competency evaluation.

INTRODUCTION

In aviation, medicine, military, and nursing, simulation-based education (SBE) has a robust historical relevance that illuminates the legitimacy and benefit of simulation education. Historical research describes simulation-based manikins and teaching strategies, with some of the first known simulators in the Song dynasty (987–1067).[1] These carefully constructed simulators were used to teach students the exact points of acupuncture. When learners placed thin, sharp acupuncture needles into the life-sized manikin, a drop of fluid would be noted at the needle tip, signifying accuracy.[1] This teaching technique provided a pathway for learners to practice and demonstrate competency. In the eighteenth century, obstetric care simulation models were focused on training midwives and medical students to deliver infants and reduce maternal mortality.[1] In nursing education, simulation-based learning began to support learners over 100 years ago with the infamous Mrs Chase. This sawdust-filled manikin provided a safe learning environment for nursing students to practice bedside care

[a] Montana State University-Mark and Robyn Jones College of Nursing, 1500 University Drive, Billings, MT 98101, USA; [b] Seattle University-College of Nursing, 901 12th Avenue, Seattle, WA 98122, USA; [c] East Tennessee State University-College of Nursing, 1276 Gilbreath Drive, PO Box 70300, Johnson City, TN 37614, USA
* Corresponding author.
E-mail address: Carrie.miller6@montana.edu

Nurs Clin N Am 59 (2024) 415–426
https://doi.org/10.1016/j.cnur.2024.02.001
0029-6465/24/© 2024 Elsevier Inc. All rights reserved.

skills, such as positioning, wound care, injections, and health assessment.[1,2] Simulation equipment has become more sophisticated and used extensively.[1,2] Advancements in various simulation technologies, including manikins, virtual reality programs, and computer-based simulations, have led to their extensive use. This diverse array of simulation equipment offers an outstanding platform for accurately assessing and developing psychomotor skills.

What is lacking in use of simulation equipment is a pathway to assess a learner's clinical reasoning and ability to gather information and apply it in an evidence-based manner. Combining psychomotor, cognitive, and affective learning requires simulation equipment, a realistic setting, and realistic clinical scenarios for learners. Simulation-based scenarios are intended to replicate real clinical situations with high interactivity and realism.[1–3] Simulation can be delivered in various ways, including in-person, screen-based, telehealth, and augmented reality. Besides using manikins, simulation-based learning is enriched by using standardized patients (SPs), simulated patients, embedded family members, task trainers, high-fidelity manikins, and gaming simulations. All encourage a concrete learning experience in a realistic learning space without risk to patients.

Over the past 60 years, advances in simulation equipment, such as Resusci Annie, are credited with improving patient outcomes.[4,5] Practicing life-saving skills using Resusci Annie begins with recognizing a problem that exists. The classic "Are you okay, are you okay?" shoulder rub of the Resusci Annie ignites whether the "patient" is in distress. The learner must decide to initiate help and begin life-saving measures or not intervene. This first action exemplifies clinical reasoning, judgment, and how the learner proceeds, followed by a psychomotor skill. This approach to education addresses 3 issues: (1) creating a learning space for learners to achieve outcomes and objectives; (2) immersing learners in a realistic and safe environment that is observed; and (3) following by a theoretically driven debrief.[4–8]

Simulation-based learning engages the learner to practice skills, take risks, and demonstrate competency. The historical background of the creation of simulation equipment illuminates the need to create simulation scenarios that can immerse a learner in a realistic clinical situation. Simulation-based scenarios intend to replicate real clinical situations.[3] Learners can use simulation-based educational experiences as an established aspect of education that requires a strong foundation of clinical reasoning, identification of unexpected or abnormal findings, and accurate technical skills. The need for clinical reasoning, skills acquisition, and creativity provides the foundation for simulation design.[3–9]

This article aims to illustrate the process of designing a simulation-based learning activity. The process is presented in 3 phases: Phase I: Creation. Simulation-based learning experiences are created due to an identified need, followed by a series of carefully orchestrated steps in logical order. Phase I contains criteria 1–6 of the Healthcare Simulation Standard of Best Practice-Simulation Design.[9] Phase II: Structure and Transparency: In the second phase, criteria 7 to 10 are presented. The focus shifts from creation to creating a transparent, theoretically driven, facilitated environment. The focus is on using evidenced-based frameworks in facilitation, prebriefing, debriefing, and evaluation. Each of these constructs in simulation-based learning can create a safe container of learning or can traumatize learners and mitigate the benefits of simulation educational learning. Phase III: Testing and Integration. The final phase in simulation design focuses on criterion 11.[9] Once a simulation scenario has been created, it must be tested or "rehearsed" before implementation into any curriculum. Each of these phases will be discussed in further detail.

PHASES OF SIMULATION DESIGN
Phase I: Creation

A systematic approach using the Healthcare Simulation Standards of Best Practice Simulation Design™ is an 11 step simulation design process (**Box 1**). Each step is evidence-based and driven by the motivation of excellence.[9,10] Designing a simulation takes time and thought. Healthcare educators and simulationists must work together to create high-quality, well-rounded, detailed simulation scenarios.[9,10] The first phase in this process is recognizing the need to develop a simulation-based scenario scaled to the learner's level. Whether in nursing school, a nurse residency program, or SBE for seasoned healthcare professionals, simulation scenarios must be engaging, relevant, and responsive to adult learning theories.[9–11]

Kolb's experiential learning theory (ELT) is a model describing how adults learn and develop knowledge through experiences. According to Kolb's theory, adults learn best when actively involved in learning and can reflect on their experiences.[11–14] The ELT model consists of 4 stages: concrete experiences, reflective observation, abstract conceptualization, and active experimentation.[11–13] In the first stage, learners have a concrete experience, such as participating in a simulation-based scenario. For example, learners in the concrete phase of Kolb's model are experiencing the prep work, prebrief, and simulation experiences. In the second stage, learners reflect on their experience and consider what worked well and what did not. This is especially prominent in the debriefing stage of simulation-based learning. Learners develop abstract concepts and theories in the third stage based on their reflections. After debriefing, it is recommended for learners to continue reflection and consider the use of journaling.[11–14] Finally, in the fourth stage, learners actively experiment with what they have learned and begin to incorporate and apply skills in clinical practice. Kolb's

---

Box 1

HEALTHCARE SIMULATION STANDARD OF BEST PRACTICE: SIMULATION DESIGN

Designing Evidence-Based Scenarios for Clinical Practice
Phase I: Creation
1. Consultation with content and simulation experts knowledgeable in simulation best practices.
2. Perform a needs assessment to provide foundational evidence for simulation-based experience.
3. Construct measurable objectives that build upon the learner's foundational knowledge.
4. Build the simulation-based experience to align modality with the objectives.
5. Design a scenario, case, or activity to provide the context.
6. Use various types of fidelity to create the required perception of realism.
Phase II: Structure and Transparency
7. Plan a learner-centered facilitative approach driven by the objectives, learners' knowledge, and level of experience, and expected outcomes.
8. Create a prebriefing plan with preparation materials and briefing to guide participant success.
9. Create a debriefing or feedback session and/or a guided reflection exercise to follow the simulation-based experience.
10. Develop a plan for evaluation of the learner and of the simulation-based experience.
    Phase III: Testing and Integration
11. Pilot test simulation-based experiences before full implantation.

From INACSL Standards Committee, Watts PI, McDermott DS, Alinier G, Charnetski M., Ludlow J, Horsley E, Meakim C & Nawathe P. Healthcare simulation standards of best practice™ simulation design. Clinical Simulation in Nursing 58; 2021:14-21. https://doi.org/10.1016/j.ecns.2021.08.009.

model provides a helpful framework for designing simulation-based educational experiences that are engaging, relevant, and responsive to adult learning theories.[11–14]

Criteria 1 and 2: Expertise and needs assessment

Conducting a thorough needs assessment across various settings is crucial to ensure relevance and effectiveness when designing simulation scenarios. This process should begin with assembling a team of content and simulation experts, each bringing valuable background and experience to the scenario design.[9] The needs assessment should focus on identifying specific areas for development or performance gaps. Needs assessment may be used when identifying the need to evaluate the competencies of both new and experienced caregivers, improving teamwork among healthcare groups, or ensuring compliance with continuing education policies. For instance, in a hospital setting, a scenario might be designed to assess the emergency response skills of medical staff, while in a primary care setting, the focus could be improving patient communication skills. By aligning the simulation design with these targeted needs, the scenarios become more impactful and directly beneficial to clinical practice.

For the exemplar scenario in this article, the content experts included nursing faculty, experienced clinical practitioners experienced in ambulatory care, and 2 simulation experts in simulation best practices. A performance gap was identified in learners lacking communication skills. The scenario was explicitly tailored for second-year prelicensure nursing students enrolled in a 4 year education program during their nutrition course. The primary consideration for the group was establishing the simulation's overarching goal, ensuring it aligns with the educational objectives of the nursing course. Considered an entry-level simulation, the primary objective was to advance the development of communication skills, which are vital for patient education in a real-world clinical environment. Offering an evidenced-based approach for students to learn and apply communication techniques directly with simulated patients early in nursing education emphasizes the importance of therapeutic communication (**Box 2**).

A goal guides the development of a simulation scenario by providing an overarching premise of the purpose of the learning activity. A goal could be related to communication, such as "*improving communication skills.*" Once the goals for the simulation scenario are determined, the course outcomes are also considered. For example, in the exemplar, one of the course outcomes is to "*Utilize the nursing process and therapeutic communication skills to communicate effectively with patients and family about nutrition-related topics, including dietary recommendations, food safety, and the role of nutrition in disease management.*"[11–14] This course outcome directly links to

---

Box 2
Simulation exemplar

Goal
- *Improving Communication Skills in second year students*

Course outcome
- *Utilize the nursing process and therapeutic communicate skills to communicate effectively with patients and family about nutrition-related topics, including dietary recommendations, food safety, and the role of nutrition in disease management.*

Simulation objectives
1. *Conduct assessments appropriate for nutritional counseling in a systematic manner.*
2. *Demonstrate effective communication, caring, cultural sensitivity, and address dietary preferences.*
3. *Practice within nursing scope of practice.*

the overall simulation scenario goal based on the needs assessment and the simulation objective.[14–17]

Criteria 3: Constructing objectives

When writing objectives, there are a few steps to consider. Evidence suggests having at most 3 to 4 simulation-specific objectives.[9,17] Every simulation-based learning experience will have general simulation objectives, such as hand hygiene or identifying the patient. The National League of Nursing Simulation Template (please see the *link:* National League of Nursing Simulation Innovation Resource Center https://www.nln. org/education/education/sirc/sirc/sirc-resources/sirc-tools-and-tips) provides a platform for simulation design and generalized simulation objectives. Each simulation objective needs to be created using SMART (specific, measurable, achievable, relevant/realistic, time-bound).[3,10,17] Simulation objectives must be appropriate to the learner's level. Placing learners in a simulation that is too advanced or expectations are not clear creates confusion, emotional trauma, and frustration. Simulations must be created where learners have been exposed to the didactic, cognitive knowledge, and opportunity to prepare for the simulation exercise.[3,8–10]

A simulation objective for the exemplar scenario is to *"Demonstrate effective communication, caring, cultural sentitivity, and address dietary preferences"* The objective is specific, with a focus on communication. The measurability comes from acts of caring and a learner's ability to demonstrate therapeutic communication. Therefore, the objective is realistic, relevant to nursing practice, and achievable during the simulation-based activity at the learners' current level. Lastly, the simulation activity will last approximately 20 minutes or when objectives have been met. Simulation scenarios should contain cues that allow learners to achieve the SBE objectives within the allotted time. Simulation objectives can be worded in a multitude of ways. However, each aspect of the simulation objective must be considered in development.[3,10,17]

Criterion 4: Modality

Once the objectives are created and mapped to link to outcomes, the next step is to determine the modality of the simulation exercises. Modality refers to the learning environment.[9] Most simulations take place in 1 of 5 modalities. Each modality needs to be considered when designing a simulation. The 5 modalities include.

1. Clinical immersion involves in-person clinical scenarios. Clinical immersion can occur in simulation centers, laboratories, or clinical settings. When clinical immersion occurs in hospitals or clinical settings at the point of care, it is commonly referred to as "in situ simulation."[9]
2. Screen-based, providing simulation scenarios involve a computer screen, mouse, joystick, or computerized platform. Commonly known as "gaming simulation," learners view recorded vignettes and make decisions regarding clinical reasoning.[9] This modality works well for simulations conducted remotely or completed in an asynchronous or synchronous learning environment.
3. Virtual reality using augmented reality technology and resources. This form of simulation is immersive and becoming more common in medical and healthcare training.[9]
4. Procedural simulation, focusing on skill acquisition or demonstrating skill competency.
5. Hybrid simulation, which includes the use of task trainers affixed to a standardized or simulated patient. An example of a hybrid simulation is using a wearable birthing simulation task trainer integrated into the simulation. Modality needs to be considered carefully and in alignment with the objectives of the simulation.[9,17]

Criterion 5: Simulation scenario creation
The steps in designing a simulation are systematic and strategic. The needs assessment guides the scenario development through goals, outcomes, objectives, and modality selection.[3,9,10,17] In creating a simulation scenario, resources may include current evidence within the literature, critical pathways, healthcare standards of practice, feedback from alums, community advisory councils, and institutional policies and procedures. The next step in the process is to design the clinical scenario. It is advised in best practices to focus on the goals from the needs assessment and then create a clinical case study that melds well. The clinical scenario needs to be relevant and realistic. Scenarios are often reflective of actual clinical situations with identifiers removed.

The scenario needs to be standardized and easily replicated. This creates an opportunity for any learner to have a similar experience. Having the patient verbalize the same cue statements at each phase standardizes the clinical situation. When creating the clinical case, consider not only the verbal consistency of scripting but also having available embedded cues, such as laboratory values, vital signs on the monitor, chart notes, and treatment results, to name a few.

Creating a well-rounded, complete case situation that is realistic, relevant, and complete is vital. In this article's exemplar, the simulation focuses on nutritional counseling and communication. The scenario background is a 46 year old female client (**Box 3**) who presents to an outpatient setting with complaints of prediabetes and dyslipidemia. She has been suffering from gastrointestinal upset, fatigue, hyperglycemia, and a recent weight gain of 20 pounds. The modality is a telehealth session with a SP trained actor. In response to fidelity, the SP is a middle-aged female individual who is similar in weight and habitus as described in the background. The SP has been trained in the medical conditions, symptoms, and expected questions a nursing professional may ask during a nutritional assessment. The SP is also trained to respond to questions with specific answers to promote standardization of all nursing students and SP interactions for this simulation-based scenario.[18] Within the chart record are available cues for learners to ask about symptoms, nutritional choices, and concerns.

When developing a case scenario, it is essential to identify critical actions. Critical actions are intended to evaluate the achievement of scenario objectives.[3,9,10,14] Facilitators and content experts who are observers of the simulation-based learning activity are looking for the essential actions to be accomplished. The critical actions are then linked to the simulation objectives and course outcomes. The essential actions in the presented scenario are to identify the patient, ask the patient the purpose of the visit, review aspects of the health history to confirm accuracy, use positive body language and therapeutic respectful communication, and demonstrate caring attitudes without judgment. All the critical actions are scaffolded to the level of the learner through didactic and laboratory activities before the simulation-based learning activity.

Box 3
Simulation background: *nutritional counseling simulation*

Fiadh Martin, 46 year old female patient who is seeking RN telehealth visit regarding concerns related to fatigue, GI upset, recent weight gain of 20 pounds in past few months. She has a primary medical diagnosis of prediabetes, hyperlipidemia, hypertension, and perimenopausal symptoms. She is seeking lifestyle change guidance and has declined to continue with lipid-regulating medication prescribed by her medical provider due to side effects.

Criterion 6: Fidelity and realism

Fidelity adds richness and realism to a simulation-based activity. Regardless of modality, fidelity is responsive to the realism of the simulation-based learning experience. When designing a simulation, where the learning takes place matters, the learning environment must reflect where the actual situation would occur. There are 3 constructs of fidelity. These include (1) environmental or physical fidelity, (2) conceptual fidelity, and (3) psychological fidelity. An example of physical fidelity is having a cardiac simulation in an emergency department, a telehealth simulation with a mental health client in crisis, or a simulation attending to an out-of-hospital birth. The physical environment creates the setting and tone of the simulation and what may be expected.[3,9,10]

The second fidelity consideration is "conceptual fidelity." In simulation-based scenarios, conceptual fidelity focuses on how things relate to one another.[3,9,10] The question must be asked whether the scenario pieces and parts link. Can the learner make sense of what is being presented? When designing the simulation exemplar, conceptual fidelity is considered with how the SP presents, the health concerns, cues, and the setting. Does having a telehealth visit to discuss generalized health concerns with a nutritional focus make sense?

Conceptual fidelity guides the learner along the learning experience and provides a platform for realism. Content experts should review conceptual fidelity. This allows for a detailed assessment of the scenario to see if there are any missing aspects and to offer insight into how to be mindful of conceptual fidelity. Thoughtfulness needs to be given to cultural influences, identity, race, and ethnicity. It is essential not to stereotype but to create scenarios that reflect the community learners will serve. In the presented exemplar, the SP is of Irish descent, immigrated to the United States in her 20s, lives with her partner, and is an artist in a local coastal community.

The third level of fidelity is psychological fidelity. When done well, learning in simulation is immersive, and learners suspend disbelief, quickly adapt to the learning situation, and conduct themselves as though they are in a real clinical setting.[9,19] Considerations must be given to lighting, sounds, alarms, family members, and distractions. These aspects provide learners the opportunity to engage in a meaningful manner.[9] In high-quality simulation-based learning, how the simulation scenario is presented sets the tone for the learners.

Phase II: Structure and Transparency

Criterion 7: Facilitation

Facilitators are responsible for setting the tone of the learning experience. The Healthcare Simulation Standards of Best Practice™ recommend formal training in simulation pedagogy.[9,19] Simulation training can be formal mentoring, conferences, workshops, or fellowships. Poor facilitation can influence student learning and create emotional distress in learners. Furthermore, a lack of proper training can impede students from meeting simulation objectives, reduce standardization of SBE, and result in student frustration and lack of engagement. In a recent editorial, Harder suggests that simulation-based learning facilitated by poorly trained individuals can lead to adverse outcomes for learners.[20] This is concerning and further exemplifies the need for appropriate, evidence-based training for all simulationists and educators involved in simulation-based pedagogy.[9,19,20] Simulation facilitators are responsible for conducting the prebrief, simulation-based activity, and the debrief. If the plan is to have more than one facilitator, a structured action plan must be in place to reduce confusion for the learners and maintain standardization. Facilitators must implement simulation-based scenarios in a learner-centered approach and incorporate evidence-based constructs.[21]

In facilitating, consideration must be given to the cultural differences among learners, knowledge level, competency, and experience in SBE. For novice learners of SBE, simulations need to be paced carefully to permit learners to adapt to the simulation learning space and expectations. Learners may appreciate the first simulation being a low-stakes, low-pressure, orientation-type simulation. With room to adjust to simulation-based learning, participants can explore simulation-based settings without the stress of a summative or high-stakes simulation experience.

Criterion 8: Preparatory Work and Prebriefing

To optimize learner success, simulation design best practices suggest structured, predetermined, and planned preparatory work for learners to complete before attending the simulation experience.[22,23] Preparatory work can vary, but the intent is to provide learners with an essential background of the case and simulation-specific objectives. In the presented exemplar, learners are expected to review a nursing-focused nutritional assessment, review assessing weight changes and implications of a significant weight change over a short time, pathophysiological concerns surrounding hyperglycemia, and provide patient education in a nonjudgmental, caring, and inclusive manner. In addition, learners receive information regarding the patient's age, medical orders, preliminary labs, and social history. The intent is to provide enough information for learners to prepare to care for an individual as they would in the clinical setting. Prep work should be a required element by learners before participating in a prebriefing session. Critical actions are not provided in preparatory work nor are anticipated concerns with the patient's condition. The script and training content of the SP needs to be provided, and the expected educational focus should be provided. These aspects will be observed during the simulation-based learning experience and used to assess whether learners meet simulation objectives.

Prebriefing sessions are critical and set the tone and expectations of the simulation-based learning experience.[22,23] The use of a preplanned prebriefing script for facilitators can be helpful for the standardization of prebriefing processes and time management. Prep work and simulation objectives can be reviewed. Questions are answered, and physiologic safety can be established. A safe learning container in simulation begins and ends with the facilitator trained in the healthcare simulation standards of evidence-based practice™.[23-25] The facilitator integrates these standards while demonstrating essential soft communication skills throughout the delivery of the simulation. These skills include friendliness, calm demeanor, inclusion, and respectful tone of voice.[23-25] The Basic Assumption provides a solid platform for learners to feel included, capable, and invested in learning (**Box 4**).

In the formative setting, learners are told that the simulation is not a test but rather an opportunity to practice skills, take risks, and normalize any feelings of awkwardness when in an unfamiliar situation.[23-26] A safe learning environment is expected for both the facilitator and the learner. This is achieved through mutual respect for the adult learning environment, allowing others to share thoughts and feelings without judgment or humiliation.[19,24-26] The learners are told their performance will not be

---

Box 4
THE BASIC ASSUMPTION

We believe that everyone participating in activities at (Insert Organization Name) is intelligent, capable, cares about doing their best, and wants to improve.

shared and is confidential. The question remains: how does the facilitator know a safe container for learning in simulation has been created? The subjective report of learners in the postsimulation evaluation feedback may reveal the presence of a safe learning container.[24,25]

Part of prebriefing is orientation to the simulation environment. The modality, rationale, and where learners can find materials are presented during orientation.[9,22] Orientation is often overlooked in simulation design. There is concern about revealing too much information to the learners. For new learners, stress can be reduced, and learning is richer if learners know where the key essential items are located, including how to communicate with providers, where vital signs will be posted, and the crucial functions of the manikin. For example, in a simulation using an SP in a tele-healthcare setting, learners will be informed where the SP will be waiting, the modality of the simulation-based experience, and how to use technical resources.

To effectively prebrief an in situ simulation in clinical practice, orienting participants to the simulation's specific simulation environment, agenda, and objectives is essential. The pre-briefing process involves facilitation implementation at the forefront once the simulation scenario has been constructed, explaining the simulation's goals, modality, rationale, and location of necessary materials. It should be tailored according to the simulation objectives, the learner's level of experience, and the unique details of the scenario, ensuring all participants are adequately prepared and informed before the simulation begins.[22,25]

For learners familiar with the simulation setting, a less detailed orientation can be considered; however, orientation needs to be a routine aspect of the simulation-based activity and responsive to the objectives, level of learner, and scenario.[22,27] After prebriefing and orientation to the room, the simulation design may include a method for assigning roles and a short breakif needed. Offering a break may let learners settle and perhaps be more mentally prepared to begin the simulation activity.

Criteria 9 and 10: Debriefing and evaluation
Simulation design must include a structured, well-planned, theoretically based debriefing framework.[7,9,10,12,20] Debriefing can include feedback or guided reflection. The primary focus of debriefing is to give space for learners to identify areas of growth and areas of strength in skills, communication, teamwork, clinical reasoning, judgment, and ability to adapt to changing or evolving clinical situations. There are numerous frameworks in simulation-based pedagogy. In simulation design, it is vital to use a debriefing framework that aligns with the level of the learner, type of simulation activity, and simulation objectives.[7,9] A debriefing framework using Socratic questions, such as Debriefing for Meaningful Learning, may prove effective for simulations focused on in-depth analysis and reflection of the simulation-based learning experience.[28] Regardless of the framework selected, training and feedback for the individual conducting the SBE is essential. As the simulation-based learning experience is being designed, considerations to the framework need to be included. Many simulation centers will collectively agree on using a single debriefing framework for consistency and standardization. Regardless of the debriefing method selected, it is critical to use a framework to its full potential and ensure facilitators are trained. Furthermore, facilitators must be educated and mentored in simulation design on effectively and correctly using the selected debriefing framework. Regardless of the framework used, it is essential to maintain a sense of psychological safety, expectations, agenda, and simulation objectives.

SBE design is a process that needs to include an evaluative component. During the simulation, the facilitator observes and evaluates the learners, whereas the learner also evaluates the simulation experience.[9,29] From first impressions to final thoughts during debriefing, an evaluative process is going on. In SBE, evaluating the simulation using a validated method is essential. Using a structured framework that includes quantitative and qualitative responses provides depth in how simulation-based experiences impact learners. Assessing simulation promotes quality and provides meaningful feedback for facilitators and stakeholders. The evaluation results are used for quality assurance, revisions, and relevance.[9]

Phase III: Testing and Integration

Criterion 11: Pilot test

Simulation design requires tremendous thought, planning, teamwork, review, revisions, and structure. Once the essential elements are in place, the final step in simulation design is to "beta" or "pilot" test the simulation activity.[9] The entire simulation-based learning experience needs a primary, detailed "dress rehearsal" to see what areas are well executed and smooth and what aspects of the simulation-based learning activity need to be revised. One factor to consider when selecting participants for the pilot testing is using alumni learners, educators, and content experts to participate in the simulation. Alumni learners have previously completed an educational program or training and can offer valuable insights based on their experience and current practices. Having the SP or embedded actor can also be beneficial. Anticipate enough time to review the prep work, practice the prebriefing session, orientation to the learning space, at least 1 full simulation round for each stage, and a debriefing session that includes not only debriefing the simulation but also debriefing and discussing the simulation activity and design itself. This information is then used to solidify or revise the simulation-based learning activity before implementation into the curriculum or program.

Pilot testing process

The pilot testing of the presented exemplar simulation involved 2 separate rounds. The second pilot test was used in response to revisions made from the first test round. The pilot test included reviewing preparatory work, prebriefing, setting the safe container, orientation to the learning space, simulation-based learning, and using a predetermined debriefing framework. The debriefing session focused on communication, cultural sensitivity, and nutritional planning.

The pilot test required 2 groups, totaling 6 nursing students who consented to participate. Each participant was at the junior level in their education. The first group of 2 students, completed the simulation in 20 minutes. In the second group, which included 4 nursing students, results indicated a longer time was needed, with revisions made to extend the simulation time to 30 minutes for groups of 4 to 5 participants.

Observation and feedback during debriefing revealed participants in the pilot testing felt they could recognize cues and respond to the standardized patients questions. Overall, the findings from the pilot test were positive. Participants suggested revising the SP script, including an embedded family member for distraction, and allowing more time for the simulation objectives to be met in a telehealth learning environment. As a result, the training for SPs now includes a focus on timekeeping and participating in the debriefing. This ensures the simulation adheres to its intended duration and remains efficient and effective for all learners. After carefully reviewing the pilot tests and feedback, the content and simulation experts determined that the simulation with revisions was sufficiently created for learners to meet simulation objectives.

SUMMARY

Healthcare educators and simulationists use various simulation-based learning experiences to meet learner needs. The development and integration of simulation scenarios is a thoughtful and systematic journey. Using best practices and evidence-based approaches provides a solid platform for this valuable teaching technique. As healthcare becomes more technologically complex and detached from the humanistic side of caregiving, simulation pedagogy can provide a meaningful foundation for learners as they deliver excellence to all they care for.

CLINICS CARE POINTS

- Prebriefing and orientation support set the tone for a psychologically safe learning environment for all participants.
- Simulation-based learning experiences create a bridge between classroom and patient care delivery.
- When debriefing, the time belongs to learners and is a time for facilitators to listen, not to teach.

DISCLOSURE

The authors have no financial or commercial conflicts of interest.

REFERENCES

1. Owen H. Early use of simulation in medical education. Simulat Healthc J Soc Med Simulat : Journal of the Society for Simulation in Healthcare 2012;7:102–16.
2. Nickerson M, Pollard MA. Mrs. Chase and her descendants: A historical view of simulation. Creativ Nurs 2010;16:101–5.
3. Waxman KT. The development of evidence-based clinical simulation scenarios: Guidelines for nurse educators. J Nurs Educ 2010;49:29–35.
4. Jones F, Passos-Neto C, Braghiroli OM. Simulation in medical education: Brief history and methodology. Principles and Practice of Clinical Research 2015;1: 56–63.
5. Piryani RM, Piryani S, Shrestha U, et al. Simulation-based education workshop: perceptions of participants. Adv Med Educ Pract 2019;547–54.
6. Davitadze M, Ooi E, Ng CY, et al. SIMBA: using Kolb's learning theory in simulation-based learning to improve participants' confidence. BMC Med Educ 2022;22(1). https://doi.org/10.1186/s12909-022-03176-2.
7. Decker S, Alinier G, Crawford SB, et al. Healthcare simulation standards of best practiceTM The debriefing process. Clin Simul Nurs 2021;58:27–32.
8. McDermott DS, Ludlow J, Horsley E, Meakim C. Healthcare simulation standards of best practiceTM prebriefing: preparation and briefing. Clin Simul Nurs 2021; 58:9–13.
9. Watts PI, McDermott DS, Alinier G, et al. Healthcare simulation standards of best practiceTM simulation design. Clin. Simul. Nurs. 2021;58:14–21.
10. Bambini D. Writing a simulation scenario: a step-by-step guide. AACN Adv Crit Care 2016;1:62–70.
11. Bobek H. Teaching strategies for online nurse practitioner physical assessment and telehealth education. Nurs Clin 2022;57(4):589–98.
12. Reierson IÅ, Haukedal TA, Hedeman H, et al. Structured debriefing: What difference does it make? Nurse Educ Pract 2017;17:104–10.

13. Murray M. The impact of interprofessional simulation on readiness for interprofessional learning in health professions students. Teach Learn Nurs 2021;16: 199–204.

14. Wijnen-Meijer M, Brandhuber T, Schneider A, et al. Implementing Kolb's experiential learning cycle by linking real experience, case-based discussion, and simulation. Journal of medical education and curricular development 2022;9.

15. Khamis N, Satava R, Alnassar S, et al. A stepwise model for simulation-based curriculum development for clinical skills, a modification of the six-step approach. Surg Endosc 2016;30:279–87.

16. Choi W, Dyens O, Chan TM, et al. Engagement and learning in simulation: recommendations of the Simnovate Engaged Learning Domain Group. BMJ Simulation and Technology Enhanced Learning 2017;3(Suppl 1):S23–32.

17. INACSL Standards Committee, Miller C, Deckers C, Jones M, et al. Healthcare simulation standards of Best Practice™ outcomes and objectives. Clinical Simulation in Nursing 2021;58:40–4.

18. Gore T, Lutz RM, Bernard R, et al. Home health simulation: Helping students meet the changing healthcare needs. J Nurs Educ Pract 2018. https://doi.org/10.5430/jnep.v9n1p27.

19. Sadd R. Ethical considerations of replacing clinical hours with simulation in undergraduate nursing education: means to an end, or an end in itself? Creativ Nurs 2023;29(2):187–91.

20. Harder N. The Silent Epidemic: Addressing the Abuse of Prelicensure Nursing Students in Simulation. Clinical Simulation in Nursing 2023;85. https://doi.org/10.1016/j.ecns.2023.101484.

21. Oyelana O, Olson J, Caine V. An evolutionary concept analysis of learner-centered teaching. Nurse Educ Today 2022;108:105187.

22. INACSL Standards Committee, McDermott DS, Ludlow J, Horsley E, et al. Healthcare simulation standards of best practice™ prebriefing: preparation and briefing. Clinical Simulation in Nursing 2021;58:9–13.

23. Tyerman J, Luctkar-Flude M, Graham L, et al. A Systematic review of health care presimulation preparation and briefing effectiveness. Clinical Simulation in Nursing 2019;27:12–25.

24. Paige J, Graham L, Sittner B. Formal training efforts to develop simulation educators: an integrative review. Simulat Healthc J Soc Med Simulat 2020;15(4): 271–81.

25. Madireddy S, Rufa EP. *Maintaining confidentiality and psychological safety in medical simulation.* https://www.ncbi.nlm.nih.gov/books/NBK559259/.

26. Rudolph J, Raemer D, Simon D. Establishing a safe container for learning in simulation: the role of the presimulation briefing. Simulat Healthc J Soc Med Simulat 2014;339–49.

27. Daniels A, Morse C, Breman R. Psychological safety in simulation-based prelicensure nursing education: A narrative review. Nurse Educat 2021;46:E99–102.

28. Dreifuerst KT. Getting started with debriefing for meaningful learning. Clinical Simulation in Nursing 2015;11(5):268–75. https://doi.org/10.1016/j.ecns.2015.01.005.

29. INACSL Standards Committee, McMahon E, Jimenez FA, Lawrence K, et al. Healthcare simulation standards of practice Evaluation of learning and performance. Clinical Simulation in Nursing 2021;58:54–6.

Simulation Modalities in Clinical Practice

Elizabeth Horsley, RN, MSMS, CHSE, CCSNE[a],*,
Jennifer Dale-Tam, RN, MSN, CNCC(c), CCSNE, CHSE[b]

KEYWORDS

• Modality • Manikin • Task trainer • In-situ • Virtual

KEY POINTS

- There are a variety of simulation modalities available to clinical simulation educators.
- The modality must be chosen to align with the learning objectives.
- Appropriate modality choice impacts the effectiveness of the simulation experience.

INTRODUCTION

The practice of simulation requires the educator/facilitator to identify the learning needs of the participants, design an appropriate activity, and select the best modality to stage the scenario/activity. Well-constructed simulation activities at their core consist of appropriate and meaningful learning objectives designed to meet the needs of a targeted learner group. The key then to effective and meaningful simulation is the choice of the simulation modality. Modality refers to the equipment platform or techniques the learners will actively engage with during the simulation activity. Modalities then are the "methods or resources used to support the simulation activity." (p.65)[1] A well-chosen modality will allow the simulation scenario or activity brought to life. The properly chosen modality will allow the learners to actively engage and ultimately achieve the learning objectives.

OVERVIEW OF SIMULATION AS AN EDUCATIONAL TECHNIQUE

On the heels of an increased commitment to patient safety in the early 2000s, clinical simulation began to gain a foothold in health professions education. Simulation emerged as an effective strategy for preparing safe and efficient health care practitioners. Academic and health care institution programs began in earnest building simulation learning laboratories and spaces and purchasing simulation equipment—most often the human patient simulator or manikin. These manikins often became a

[a] St Catharines, PO Box 640, Vineland, Ontario L0R2C0, Canada; [b] The Ottawa Hospital, 501 Smyth Road, Ottawa, Ontario K1H 8L6, Canada
* Corresponding author. PO Box 640, Vineland, Ontario L0R2C0, Canada.
E-mail address: ehorsleysimulation@gmail.com

Nurs Clin N Am 59 (2024) 427–436
https://doi.org/10.1016/j.cnur.2024.02.009
0029-6465/24/© 2024 Elsevier Inc. All rights reserved.
nursing.theclinics.com

showcase item for the institution as well as being educational workhorse. As the decades progressed, and simulation theory and pedagogy evolved, more and varied simulation modalities gained a foothold. Although manikins had their place, other modalities were found to be more effective, depending on the learning objectives of the experience. Emerging modalities ranged from task trainers to table-top activities to the recent boon in virtual experiences from screen-based to immersion via headset.

An effective simulation program need not always involve costly technology or high-tech gadgetry. Simulation is often associated with high-tech patient manikin type units or standardized patients who are actors trained to portray a specific condition or situation. The simulation umbrella, however, also encompasses the vast array of skill-based training initiatives from arms for practicing blood draws to robotic surgical simulators. A well thought out session with focused practice on opening a sterile field and inserting a foley catheter is certainly a simulation-based educational experience. Simulation does not have to have, as they say, all "the bells and whistles." Regardless of the advances in modality technology and capabilities, the fact remains that high-quality simulation design requires meaningful thought as to the most appropriate simulation modality. The latest innovations in technology in a modality will not necessarily yield the best educational results. The onus remains on the educator to match the anticipated learning outcomes and objectives with the most appropriate modality.

This paper explores common simulation modalities that simulation educators can implement in clinical or academic settings. This listing is by no means exhaustive of all the potential choices of modalities available currently. The modalities discussed were chosen by the authors who are both experienced hospital-based simulation specialists.

MODALITIES
Manikin-Based Simulation

Who: educators who began using simulation during the past 2 decades more than likely had their first experiences with manikins. As simulation learning laboratories and spaces began to be developed in health professions schools, the manikins were often the first and most common modality to appear. Although there are numerous modality options available today, and the advancements in technology are rapid, manikins most certainly will always have a place in the wide and every growing simulation world.

What: manikins can represent a full or partial body (the torso) of a patient within a simulation-based educational activity. Manikins can have varying levels of technology with respect to how their vital signs and other physiologic parameters are controlled. Are they controlled remotely or by a handheld unit? Do they require an air compressor to allow for chest rise and fall? Can the manikin show signs of diaphoresis or cyanosis? Manikins vary in their level of realism ranging from basic units that are a simple representation of a patient to units that have a realistic skin texture, blinking eyes, pupillary responses, or ability to inject fluids. Manikins are available to represent patients across the lifespan from premature infants to school-age children to geriatric adults (**Fig. 1**).

A discussion of manikins is an appropriate place to make the distinction between two oft-used terms in simulation: technology and fidelity. Although the terms are often used interchangeably, there is a definitive distinction between the two. Technology refers to qualities and capabilities of the manikin, whereas fidelity "refers to the realism of the entire scenario" (p.184).[2] It is entirely possible for a simulation experience to use the highest level of technology available, yet the scenario may be completely unrealistic or improbable, thus rendering it low fidelity.

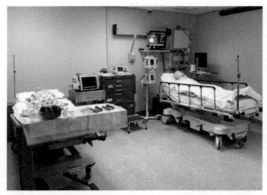

Fig. 1. Adult and pediatric manikins.

Where: perhaps the only limitations on the use of manikins are the costs (initial purchase and maintenance and consumables) and the need for adequate space for a full, simulated human body to be housed. For smaller or resource-challenged centers, there are upper-body torso manikins available, which can provide some of the benefits of the full-body patient but are more portable and require less space.

Why: manikins are used in "a scenario where a central element of the scenario, often the patient, is a full-body manikin" (p.30).[3] These types of scenarios may involve performing several skills that just would not be feasible (or ethical) on a standardized or simulated patient such as chest compressions, defibrillation, or the insertion of a nasogastric tube. Simulations with objectives for therapeutic communication or interpersonal skills needed between patient and provider are generally not the best use of a manikin. Although some manikins have the ability to speak preprogrammed statements for intensive patient engagement, an actual simulated patient would be a better choice.

When: manikins can be costly and cumbersome; however they can be used in a multitude of simulations and allow for multiple learners and repetitive practice. The use of the manikin depends on objectives of the scenario and what skills and abilities to be performed by the learners.

How: the scenario will be designed, keeping in mind that the manikin will be representing the patient. How should the manikin present? If communication is required, does the scenario allow for a family member or significant person to "speak for" the manikin patient? Is there any limitation with the available manikin? Some manikins can be defibrillated or have fluids infused. Be aware of the capabilities and limitations of the manikin as the scenario is being developed. Also, manikins are not limited to just being a patient in a bed. Manikins can be dressed in street clothes and strategically placed—for example, in a hospital cafeteria or a parking lot—for maximum effectiveness of a scenario around a sudden cardiac arrest. Moulage can be applied to manikins, for example, burns or oozing wounds, to enhance the realism of a scenario. The potential for manikin-based simulation is only limited by the creativity of the simulation educators (**Fig. 2**)!

Task Trainers

What: a task trainer is a tool or device designed specifically to train on the essential elements of a procedure or skill. It usually represents a part of the human body. Some task trainers provide mechanical or electronic feedback to the learner.[4] Sometimes they are referred to as part-task trainers. Task trainers can be as simple using an

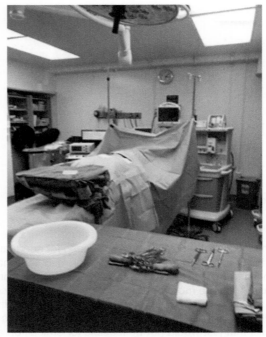

Fig. 2. Manikin draped and ready for the operating room.

orange to practice intramuscular injections to a torso to practice nasogastric tube insertion to a central venous access device manikin to practice accessing central lines.

Who: task trainers can be used by any health care educator but do require knowledge on proper setup of the device and ongoing maintenance. If used as part of a hybrid simulation or full-scale simulation the session should be facilitated by an educator who is trained to do so.[5]

Where: task trainers can be used anywhere there is space to conduct the session. They may be housed in formal simulation spaces to classrooms to carts that are easily portable and can be taken wherever a skill refresher is required.

Why: task trainers are used to practice focused skills without the added cognitive load of a full-scale simulation. It allows learners to develop mastery through repetitive deliberate practice with mechanisms of feedback. Many times, task trainers are used as a preparation to full-scale simulation, which is in alignment with the best practices of health care simulation.[6]

How: laboratory instructors can deliver sessions 1:1 with students or in a large group where learners rotate through various skill stations with the instructor roaming station to station to provide feedback. If learners are left to practice skills on a task trainer on their own, there must be a method of feedback so that poor habits are not repeated. A rubric or skills checklist can be used to provide peer to peer feedback for task trainers that do not have mechanisms of feedback as part of their design.

Case-Based Discussion

What: case-based discussion is a form of low fidelity simulation. It is regarded as a participatory teaching-learning approach that encourages participants to learn actively and reflectively to sharpen their critical thinking and problem-solving abilities.[7] It is a form of problem-based learning where learners work through a scenario presented to them with questions or prompts to cue their thought processes. Sometimes case-based discussion is referred to as "tabletop simulation" or role play when there is more active involvement of learners in taking roles within the case.

Who: case-based discussion has been used by many health professions. It has been found to be used as early as 1912 in medical education.[8] Regarding nursing, it has primarily been used in academia to link theory to practice but has gained traction in practice environments as part of the onboarding process for nurses to new clinical environments or as part of professional development programs. Nurse educators, simulation educators, clinical instructors, and nurse preceptors and preceptees can easily implement this method of reflective and engaging education.

Where: case-based learning can be used in the classroom to engage learners in any aspect of knowledge they are learning. Other applications include the following:

- In the post conference session after a nursing student clinical placement;
- As an in-service on a clinical nursing unit or clinic facilitated by a nurse educator with unit/clinic staff;
- A form of "mental" rehearsal between a nurse preceptor and nursing student or new staff member before doing a clinical procedure or skill;
- Part of an independent ongoing professional development learning plan for a nurse.

Why: through the utilization of realistic clinical scenarios, case-based discussion aims to prepare health practitioners for clinical practice. Through the application of knowledge to instances and the use of inquiry-based learning techniques, it connects theory to practice.[7] Case-based discussion requires little to no resources to implement.

How: cases are usually based on a real clinical patient or situation that has been deidentified to maintain confidentiality. In the classroom the case can be presented on a slide presentation followed by open-ended questions to prompt discussion. In a clinical space it can be presented on paper or verbally by the educator with the learner and/or listened to followed by prompts or question for discussion.

An effective method to stimulate further knowledge acquisition and critical thinking is to use an "unfolding case study." A short case stem is provided to the learner with one to two questions to stimulate discussion and answers. As answers are solidified and assessment findings are uncovered by the learners, more of the case is revealed small bits at a time with questions to prompt further thinking and answers. This method of case-based discussion replicates real-world progression of patient care but is low resource and a simple method to implement.

Hybrid Simulation

What: hybrid simulations involve the pairing of two (or more) simulation modalities. Most commonly, part-task trainers are paired with simulated patients. A simulated patient can be gowned and in a hospital bed with a foley catheter training model placed in their perineal area. This allows the learner to perform the skill of catheterization while also communicating with the patient. Another great use of this type of pairing is a simulated patient representing a labouring mother with a birthing pelvis placed in front of the patient's abdomen. Again, the learners can engage with the tasks of delivery while having to communicate with the patient and her support people. In another instance, a scenario may begin with a simulated patient who presents to an emergency department and is interviewed by staff. This "patient" may then lose consciousness, and the scenario would move over to a manikin to complete more invasive aspects of care.

Who: hybrid can be effectively used in any simulation program that has the necessary equipment and people to implement and coordinate hybrid activities. Those involved in these types of simulation activities need to have competence in training and preparing simulated patients and in the use of the task trainer.

Where: hybrid simulations can work in a laboratory, classroom or in-situ setting.

Why: combining modalities allows for more realism in that learners need to engage and communicate with the patient while carrying out the required tasks. The learners now need to speak with the patient while initiating the intravenous line or suturing the laceration.

How: currently, there are several "wearable products" on the market that can be placed on a simulated patient (or a mannequin to heighten its functionality). In designing the simulation-based activity, the objectives can reflect the behavioral/skills domain and the affective/attitudinal domains.

Simulated/Standardized Patients

What: also known as "actor, embedded participant, role player, simulated person, standardized patient" (p.43).[4] These are people who are trained to accurately and realistically portray a patient, health care practitioner, or a family member. Simulated/standardized patients have received focused training on their character and are trained to be extremely realistic and provide a standardized performance with every learner encounter. A simulation may not have the access or resources to hire "simulated/standardized patients" and may choose to have faculty, staff, or other learners role play. The caveat here is that the role players have a well-developed script and a solid understanding of their role for maximum effectiveness.

Who: fully, properly trained and prepared simulated patients can be a timely and costly endeavor. Their use should be reserved for instances in which having the ability to interact and engage is paramount to achieving the learning objectives such as high-stakes evaluations.

Where: simulated patients may be used in simulation laboratory settings or classrooms. In certain instances, they may be beneficial to an in-situ scenario. Their usage will depend on the learning objectives and outcomes of the experience.

Why: the use of a real-life participant allows learners to have maximum levels of engagement. As well, simulated patients may be used in testing situations such as the Objective Structure Clinical Examinations (OSCEs) where it is of utmost importance to have a standardized performance from patients. In an OSCE situation simulated patients can be trained to provide specific feedback to learners.

How: the decision to incorporate simulated patients into a simulation-based activity begins with the learning objectives. Is this activity for a specific form of communication? The scenario should be scripted so the SP is able to provide the desired responses or information when engaging with the learner. If the simulated patients are to be used for evaluation purposes, this requires a process of developing validated and reliable scenarios and assessment tools.

Virtual Simulation

What: virtual simulation is a broad concept that encompasses computer or screen-based applications of simulation. There are no agreed on formal definitions of what virtual simulation is. These definitions include, but are not limited to, the following:

- Virtual reality simulation with full immersion of the participant in the scenario using googles and haptic devices;
- Augmented reality simulation where artificial information is superimposed on real-world objects[4];
- Serious games or virtual simulation games that use game-based theory and concepts to solve a real-world problem using a computer as the mode of delivery of the simulation.

Verkuyl and colleagues provide an excellent chart in their e-book Virtual Simulation: An Educator's Toolkit illustrating the types of virtual simulation (**Fig. 3**).

Who: the COVID-19 pandemic saw an increase in the use of virtual simulations. Various forms of virtual simulation were used to replace or augment limited clinical placements for nursing students. These simulations were done with a nurse educator present to facilitate the scenario and debriefing in real time or asynchronously where a nursing student worked through a simulation scenario then reflect on their experience using a debriefing rubric. When facilitated by a nurse educator, similar to all other modalities of simulation, the nurse educator needs to be competent in the use of the technology and be trained on how to facilitate simulation. A consideration is that fully immersive virtual simulation may not be appropriate for individuals with vestibular issues.

Where: virtual simulation can be used over large geographic distances allowing for greater access for individuals in remote areas to participate in a simulation such as telesimulation (see **Fig. 3**).[9] When immersive virtual simulation is used with google and haptic devices this can be done in any teaching room that is available in a clinical setting.

How: virtual simulation requires access to information technology infrastructure, computers, and associated equipment such as keyboards, screen, and a mouse so the participant can engage with the simulation. In countries or organizations that are low-resourced virtual simulation may not be a good option.

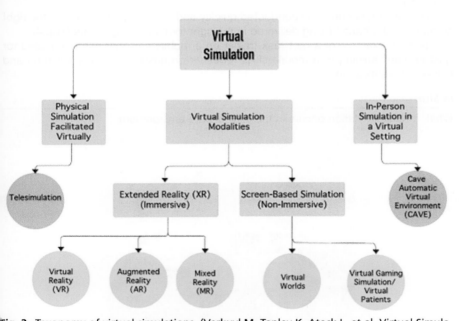

Fig. 3. Taxonomy of virtual simulations. (Verkuyl M, Taplay K, Atack L, et al. Virtual Simulation: An Educator's Toolkit.; 2022.)

Why: virtual simulation can be used as a stand-alone technique where participants apply knowledge and/or skills previously learned. In the current climate of simulation, virtual simulations, such as virtual simulation games, are used in many instances as prelearning requisite to in-person simulation where a manikin or simulated person is used as the modality.

APPLICATION
Just-in-Time

What: just-in-time simulation refers to skill training conducted immediately before a real-time, real patient intervention. Often this involves the use of a task trainer (see **Fig. 3**) that is placed on some kind of mobile cart and can be transported to the appropriate location.

Who: often, learners may progress through the steps of deliberate practice and mastery learning and demonstrate competency in a skill set. The problem lies in the inability to perform the skills regularly enough to maintain a competency level of performance. Just-in-time training allows for refresher training for staff before performing a new or rarely performed procedure.

Where: usually these trainings occur near the actual locale. Just-in-time may also be described as a "rolling refresher course."

Why: just-in-time allows for immediate practice in response to an identified need. Ideally, with just-in-time training, the learner has a basic level of skill and knowledge of the procedure, and the just-in-time session provides a rapid refresher. For example, a new hire registered nurse (RN) may have limited experience with central line dressing changes. Just before completing this task on a patient, a setup with a central line task trainer would be brought near the patient care area, and the novice nurse would have a chance to perform the skill with guidance and coaching from a more experienced practitioner.

How: learning needs to be conducted quickly and efficiently—in essence, the right amount of information being delivered in the right form at the right time (**Fig. 4**).

This is an example of a part-task trainer on a mobile cart that has been used for "just-in-time" training or a mobile skills refresher on nasogastric tube insertion and placement verification.

In-Situ

What: in-situ simulation occurs in the clinical care environment.

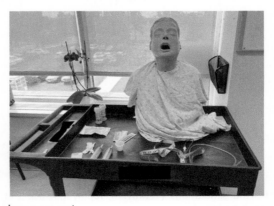

Fig. 4. Part-task trainer on a cart.

Who: in-situ simulation will include a part of the health care team, such as practicing nurses or the entire health care team including physicians, nurses, respiratory therapists, and other health professions along with the simulation educator. If using a complex manikin that replicates physiologic response through computer program, it is helpful to have additional help to operate the manikin while the simulation educator can focus on how the scenario unfolds and the debriefing afterward.

Where: it can occur in the patient care space or in an area that is adjacent to the care space such as a conference room. Sometimes this is referred to as an on-site simulation.[10]

Why: the modality used depends on the learning objectives of the session. If the learning objectives are focused on resuscitation and team function a manikin would be used. If the learning objective is regarding communication with the patient, a simulated patient would be the best fit. If communication with the patient *and* completing a medical procedure on the patient are the learning objectives, a hybrid simulation would be best using a part-task trainer and simulated patient.

How: The modality that is selected for the in-situ simulation needs to be easily transportable particularly if the simulation educator is working alone. Other considerations are method of transport, such as a stretcher or wheelchair, and the space that the simulation will occur in. Consideration of time for set up of the selected modality before the simulation taking place needs to occur, especially if in a patient care space.

NEW HIRE ORIENTATION

What: when using simulation as part of new hire orientation the modalities that are selected should be scaffolded to provide increasing complexity in application of knowledge and skills of the participants. Nurses need to come with knowledge that was previously learned to apply in the simulation session to be in alignment with best practices.[11] The knowledge may be delivered using lectures, independent learning, or asynchronous learning using a learning management system.

Who: the participants' level of experience should be considered. The more novice the nurse, the simpler the modality to start with. The more complex modalities of simulation may increase the cognitive load of the learner, thereby overwhelming the learner's ability to engage with the simulation to their full potential.

Where: within the orientation program, simulation fits well once nurses have been able to meet with the educator and spend time developing relationships with their peers. On the first day of orientation simpler modalities such as case-based discussion could be used followed by increased modality complexity in the next days or weeks.

Why: simulation-based orientations have the potential to retain health care staff and decrease orientation time.[10] Most undergraduate nursing programs incorporate simulation-based education as part of the learning process; nurses new to the profession have come to expect it to be part of their workplace learning options. Using a scaffolding approach when selecting the modality will assist in the success of the orientation program.

How: see **Fig. 5** for a suggested approach to scaffolding simulation modalities to be used in an orientation program.

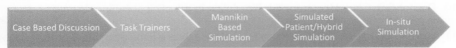

Fig. 5. Increasing modality complexity of knowledge and skills required of participants.

SUMMARY

Modality in simulation is the use of various simulation tools, techniques, or methods throughout a training session. Diverse types of modalities from case-based discussion to virtual to manikin-based simulation have been discussed, along with related applications of the various modalities. Appropriate selection of the modality to match the learning objectives is of the utmost importance to ensure a high-quality simulation-based education session along with knowledge and functional task alignment. The educator using the modality needs to be competent in its use along with training in the area of facilitation.[6]

CLINICS CARE POINTS

- Choice of modality considers learning objectives, level of learner, and resources available to the facilitator.
- Educators/facilitators must be competent in facilitating simulation.

DISCLOSURE

The authors have nothing to disclose.

REFERENCES

1. Cole R, Flenady T, Heaton L. High fidelity simulation modalities in preregistration nurse education programs: a scoping review. Clinical Simulation in Nursing 2023;80:64–86.
2. Slone FL, Lampotang S. Mannequins: terminology, selection, and usage. In: Palaganas JC, Maxworthy JC, Epps CA, et al, editors. Defining excellence in simulation programs. Philadelphia: Wolters Kluwer Health; 2015. p. 183–98.
3. Charnetski MD. Simulation methodologies. In: Crawford SB, Baily LW, Stormy MM, editors. Comprehensive healthcare simulation: operations, technology, and innovative practice. Cham (Switzerland): Springer International Publishing; 2019. p. 27–46.
4. Lioce L, Lopreiato J, Downing D, et al, Concepts Working Group. Healthcare simulation dictionary. Rockville (MD): Agency for Healthcare Research and Quality; 2020. p. 2020, 20-0019.
5. Hallmark B, Brown M, Peterson DT, et al. Healthcare Simulation Standards of Best PracticeTM Professional Development. Clin Simul Nurs 2021;58:5–8.
6. Persico L, Belle A, DiGregorio H, et al. Healthcare Simulation Standards of Best PracticeTM Facilitation. Clin Simul Nurs 2021;58:22–6.
7. Li S, Ye X, Chen W. Practice and effectiveness of "nursing case-based learning" course on nursing student's critical thinking ability: A comparative study. Nurse Educ Pract 2019;36(759):91–6.
8. McLean SF. Case-Based Learning and its Application in Medical and Health-Care Fields: A Review of Worldwide Literature. J Med Educ Curric Dev 2016;3. https://doi.org/10.4137/jmecd.s20377. JMECD.S20377.
9. Verkuyl M, Taplay K, Atack L, et al. Virtual simulation: an Educator's Toolkit; 2022. Available at: https://ecampusontario.pressbooks.pub/vlsvstoolkit/.
10. Posner GD, Clark ML, Grant VJ. Simulation in the clinical setting: towards a standard lexicon. Adv Simul 2017;2(1):1–5.
11. McDermott DS, Ludlow J, Horsley E, et al. Healthcare Simulation Standards of Best PracticeTM Prebriefing: Preparation and Briefing. Clin Simul Nurs 2021;58:9–13.

Using Simulation to Improve Communication Skills

Crystel L. Farina, PhD, RN, CNE, CHS-E[a],*,
Jasline Moreno, MSN, RN, CHSE-A, CNE[b],
Tonya Schneidereith, PhD, MBA, CRNP, PPCNP-BC, CPNP-AC, CNE, CHSE-A, ANEF, FSSH[c]

KEYWORDS

- Communication • Simulation • Teaching • Incivility • Diversity • Virtual patients
- Nursing

KEY POINTS

- Teaching communication skills is necessary in a healthcare environment.
- Simulation-based education is a strategy to enhance communication skills.
- Practicing communication during simulation supports self-reflection and uncovering biases that potentially affect patient outcomes.

INTRODUCTION

Communication is a fundamental skill for all health professionals. Relaying information between members of the healthcare team, patients, and families is needed to achieve positive patient outcomes.[1] According to Janagama and colleagues,[2] and the National Academy of Medicine (NAM),[3] in their landmark report, approximately 80% of all medical errors can be attributed to ineffective communication among the healthcare team and inadequate or confusing communication with patients and their families.[2,3]

Miscommunication is a healthcare safety issue with significant financial implications. Data show medication-related hours cost $42 billion and $12 billion of that can be attributed to ineffective communication.[2–5,] These alarming data demonstrate a need for enhanced communication education for all health professionals. This chapter focuses on simulation as a strategy for teaching essential communication skills.

Simulation, a pedagogical strategy, continues to evolve in nursing education. It uses healthcare environments, virtual reality (VR), and standardized participants to create

[a] Department of Nursing, George Washington University School of Nursing, 45085 University Drive, Ashburn, VA 20147, USA; [b] Maryland Clinical Resource Consortium, Montgomery College, 7600 Takoma Avenue, Takoma Park, MD 20912, USA; [c] SIMPL Simulation, LLC 10807 Falls Road, 694, Brooklandville, MD 21022, USA
* Corresponding author.
E-mail address: cfarina@gwu.edu

Nurs Clin N Am 59 (2024) 437–448
https://doi.org/10.1016/j.cnur.2024.02.007
0029-6465/24/© 2024 Elsevier Inc. All rights reserved.
nursing.theclinics.com

safe spaces for learners. Simulation-based experiences (SBEs) have become an effective strategy to enhance communication among members of the healthcare team, patients, and families. SBEs encourage teamwork and collaboration, foster effective communication, and improve patient outcomes.[6] Simulation scenarios used to educate healthcare professionals allow communication errors to happen in a psychologically safe learning environment without risk to patients. Debriefing the communication in the scenarios has the potential to improve communication in actual care settings.

TEACHING COMMUNICATION

Numerous reports from the NAM and the Agency for Healthcare Research and Quality (AHRQ) indicate that patient safety and healthcare outcomes continue to be an issue in the United States.[7,8] Teaching communication is a key factor to improving safety and patient outcomes, including education related to patients, families, teams, conflict, incivility, and diverse populations. How the healthcare team communicates with each other, patients, and families has an impact on the exposure to potential harms, vulnerabilities, and healthcare disparities.[8]

Communication skills are part of humanistic literacy.[9] The communication process needs senders, messages, receivers, and feedback.[10] It is a closed loop process (**Fig. 1**). However, obstruction of closed loop communication happens due to emotions, feelings, interpretation, and previous schema.[11] Although nurses and healthcare team members may think that their message is clear, the meaning is based on interpretation by the receiver. Communication errors are likely to happen when the loop is broken or not closed, the receiver is not fully listening, the sender's output is unclear, or there is a turbulent receiver/sender relationship.[8]

Dialogue may seem clear and concise, and yet nonverbal cues send a different message that leads to misunderstandings and misperceptions of the message and feedback. These dynamics affect the communication relationship and the interpretation of the message. Nurse–physician, nurse–patient–physician, and nurse–family communications have been contributors of healthcare mishaps.[8]

Nursing faculty may find it difficult to teach communication during SBEs due to the multitude of contexts in which the communication is experienced.[12] It is not enough to

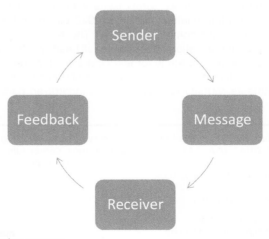

Fig. 1. Communication process.

teach how to communicate; there is a need to teach communication in multiple contexts for which communication skills and styles are needed. The following sections address concepts and contexts included in teaching communication for patients, families, teams, conflict, incivility, and diverse populations.

Patient Teaching

Nurse–patient communication is crucial to establishing a therapeutic relationship.[13] Building rapport involves developing trust, empathy, and openness with patients, which contributes to better patient outcomes and overall satisfaction. Communicating patient education, conditions, treatments, and self-care is essential for nurses.[13,14] By fostering clear and empathetic communication, nurses help patients better understand their healthcare needs and strengthen opportunities to make informed decisions.

Learners report that simulation enhances understanding of verbal and nonverbal communication during patient encounters and discharge teaching scenarios.[15] Simulation in conjunction with online learning modules have proved to be a successful strategy for educating nurses about effective discharge teaching, leading to reductions in hospital readmissions.[16] High-fidelity simulation and use of standardized patients further reinforce the significance of successful discharge and patient teaching, allowing for seamless transfer to the clinical setting[15,17,36] (**Box 1**).

Team Communication

Team communication plays a vital role in patient safety, improving overall quality care, and healthcare outcomes.[6] In 2005, AHRQ[7] and the US Department of Defense developed TeamSTEPPS to improve communication among healthcare teams.[7] Incorporation of TeamSTEPPS into interprofessional education (IPE) curricula shows significant improvement in healthcare communication.[18] Teaching communication in nursing programs is essential to support the integral role of the nurse in direct patient care.[19] Nurses must learn effective communication with each other and members of the healthcare team. SBE encourages teamwork and collaboration, fostering interdisciplinary communication, and improved patient outcomes (**Box 2**).

Simulation-based IPE can be used to teach interprofessional communication.[20] Mahmood and colleagues[21] evaluated an interprofessional simulation education module for undergraduate medical and nursing students using the TeamSTEPPS framework. Findings indicated a positive impact on communication between medical and nursing students. Tools including the communication acronym ISBAR (Introduction, Situation, Background, Assessment, and Recommendation) have been successfully

---

Box 1
Concepts for teaching communication

1. Therapeutic communication

2. Patient/family education

3. Closed loop communication

4. Interprofessional communication

5. Difficult conversations

6. Patient reports (ISBAR)

7. Incivility and conflict resolution

Box 2
Examples of simulation scenarios to practice communication during high-stress events

- Surgical procedures
- Labor and delivery
- Cardiac/respiratory arrest
- Trauma/emergency
- Pandemic/disasters
- Pediatric emergencies

---

used to teach nurse–physician communication. The development of valid and reliable rubrics, as demonstrated by Foronda and colleagues,[22] allows for standardized assessment of ISBAR's effectiveness. Kukko and colleagues[23] posits that SBE provides an opportunity for practicing team interactions in an authentic environment that is safe and enhances development of interpersonal communication competency.

Conflict Resolution

SBE is a valuable tool for teaching management of challenging situations, including medication errors, delegation, and bullying, by emphasizing the importance of communication[24] (**Table 1**). In a recent study Sowko and colleagues[23] innovatively developed trigger videos depicting real-life scenarios and used them during small group learning sessions. Learners were provided an immersive experience that evoked genuine emotions when facing difficult situations. Following the video exposure, learners were encouraged to engage in dialogue, collaboratively seeking resolutions to the conflicts presented.[25]

Medical Errors

Disclosing medical errors to patients and families is another complex skill that healthcare teams need to master. Ottis and colleagues[6] used standardized family members (SFMs) in an interprofessional simulation to teach healthcare teams effective communication to disclose errors. The SFMs used the Communication Assessment Tool–Team

---

Table 1
Simulation scenarios to manage difficult conversations

Difficult Conversation	Topic
1. Medication errors	• Disclosing an error to patients and families • Reporting errors to physicians or nursing supervisors
2. Incivility	• Confronting a coworker about uncivil behaviors • Managing incivility with patients and families
3. Relaying bad news	• Listening while a patient expresses their concerns and fears • Talking with patients and families about end-of-life needs
4. Diversity	• Managing microaggressions • Conversing when there is a language barrier • Talking with patients and families of different cultures and backgrounds
5. Body language	• Recognizing aggressive body language • Practicing a relaxed and listening body posture

(CAT-T) consisting of observable behaviors to provide feedback to learners. Ottis and colleagues[6] demonstrated incorporating the CAT-T as an important component for interprofessional teams to receive feedback and improve communication skills. Practice settings have opportunities for healthcare professionals to practice communicating medical errors during team meetings and professional development sessions. Using a team approach to this communication has the potential to decrease litigation, as patients and families understand the error, process of mitigation, and care provided now that the error has occurred.

Incivility Conflicts

Hierarchical situations among team members and patients can stilt communication due to potential rank conflicts that may create sender-receiver discomfort. For example, nurses having ideas to potentially improve patient care may perceive intimidation by other members of the healthcare team, therefore limiting their comfort sharing ideas. The voice of the hierarchy can contribute to this.[26] Listening to diverse thoughts and ideas from all levels of healthcare can improve patient outcomes and healthcare systems.[26]

Incivility and hostility in the workplace are contributing factors for new nurses leaving the profession.[27] Professional nurses play a role in teaching colleagues how to manage conflict and incivility. Expressing feelings of bullying and incivility can be difficult when the perceived bullying is coming from a person who has power over their success. According to Howard and Embree,[27] communication and confrontation of bullying and incivility are needed to provide a safe positive work environment. Educating nurses to address incivility and bullying in a professional, positive manner during SBE can improve conflict management and nurse retention.[27]

Communication with Family Members

Simulating care of patients with family members present is an added challenge for learners. The inclusion of family in SBE increases the complexity of the experience and ensures that nurses manage patient privacy when sharing information, provide detailed teaching, and continue therapeutic and professional communication during adverse interactions. Additionally, the integration of SBE is crucial for teaching effective communication skills in the context of palliative care. Markiewicz and colleagues[28] suggests that SBE can complement existing curricula like the End-of-Life Nursing Education Consortium by incorporating specific training on palliative communication. Moreover, the use of online communication training modules has demonstrated positive effects on nurses' attitudes, knowledge, and skills when communicating with caregivers of patients with cancer,[29] and this highlights the potential of integrating online resources to enhance education and provide practice opportunities to promote effective communication in challenging healthcare contexts. Virtual SBE has emerged as an effective modality for teaching how to effectively communicate with patients and families regarding difficult topics such as bad news surrounding death and dying.[30]

There is a need for consistent meaningful feedback to the learner supporting their communication development and skills.[31] Evaluation rubrics and instruments, such as the CAT-T30 and Interprofessional ISBAR Communication Rubric,[23] provide nurses consistent, standardized mechanisms providing guidance and support for communication skill progression.[31]

Communication with Diverse Populations

English as a second language, nonnative English speakers, and biases can affect patient safety and the patient's ability to understand individual care needs. Nonnative English speakers often hesitate to seek healthcare until the need is urgent. Not only is language a barrier to communication but culture of the US healthcare system can be frightening to those who lack understanding.[26,32] Breakdowns in communication, assumptions, and misunderstandings plague healthcare settings and are linked to medication, medical, and patient compliance errors.[26] Women of minority populations are at greater risk for healthcare–related errors due to communication mishaps.[33] The use of interpreters and language interpreting resources is needed to ensure correct communication with patients, families, and members of the healthcare team.[33] The nursing profession needs support for the success of English-as-an-Additional-Language nurses to address health disparities among minority nursing groups effectively.

Responsibility for ensuring that patients and families feel respected and safe receiving healthcare rests with all healthcare professionals. The LGBTQ+ community struggles to find respectful and supportive nurses and providers.[34] Additionally, nurses and healthcare professionals continue to be inadequately educated to manage care in LGBTQ+ populations.[34] Patients from diverse gender minority groups have had challenging interactions with healthcare systems that resulted in negative patient outcomes.[35] There is a need for healthcare professionals to be proactive, educated, and up-to-date about terminology, ensuring communication is clear, supportive, and encourages members of the LGBTQ+ community to feel comfortable communicating all care needs. Negative interactions have led patients to distrust care providers, expect discrimination, and/or avoid seeking help with healthcare concerns.[35] Healthcare professionals have a responsibility to advocate for those who are unable to advocate for themselves.

Nursing and Medicine programs need opportunities for learners to practice communication with diverse vulnerable populations in psychologically safe settings. However, discussions about care needs of the LGBTQ+ community can uncover unknown attitudes and biases of learners and catch faculty unprepared for meaningful dialogue.[36] Faculty preparation is essential to have psychologically safe debriefing discussions with learners who have diverse opinions about LGBTQ+ individuals. Practicing communication skills with diverse vulnerable populations in the simulation environment provides opportunities for self-reflection about performance, communication styles, and biases (**Table 2**). The best way to change personal biases is to become aware of them. Simulation is a psychologically safe environment to implement those changes.[35,36]

Diverse backgrounds and previous experiences can influence communication skills.[37] In an increasingly diverse world, it is crucial to ensure diversity among healthcare providers, and this necessitates recruitment, retention, and graduation of diverse populations into healthcare professions. Standardized patient or simulated patient or standardized participant (SP) simulation has been identified as a valuable tool for facilitating positive outcomes for diverse learners.[37] According to a study conducted by King and colleagues,[37] participating in SP simulations led to a significant improvement in personal communication skills with patients and families, enabling the development of therapeutic relationships.

Table 2	
Simulation scenario activities to enhance communication with diverse populations	
English as a Second Language	• Using language resources/interpreters • Educating patients about US healthcare culture • Learning about cultures of others
LGBTQ+ Communities	• Communicating sexual health and reproductive needs • Establishing patient rapport • Recognizing biases

COMPLICATIONS OF COMMUNICATION

Healthcare teams use communication to relay information about patient care, treatments, diagnostic outcomes, care plans, and patient education. It is vital that learners have an opportunity to practice these communication pathways to ensure integration of the necessary knowledge, skills, and attitudes. Nurse–physician communication has historically been considered turbulent. However, the use of SBE and IPE encourages the practice of nurse–physician communication, potentially decreasing communication problems.

Communication during patient hand-off can also affect patient safety.[38] According to Janagama and colleagues,[2] the patient hand-off contributes to 80% of serious medical errors in acute care settings. Unfortunately, even though nurses practice giving report using ISBAR, key information is often missed that can be detrimental to patient outcomes. Miscommunication or missing information can happen anytime in the hand-off, from prehospital through the discharge process.[2] IPE practicing the patient hand-off can increase comfort with ISBAR communication techniques and ensure delivery of correct information.[38–40]

Electronic health record documentation is a form of communication that can affect patient outcomes. Miscommunication of information such as vital signs or assessment data can lead to improper medications, nonessential diagnostic studies, and missed symptoms of medical and medicine-related complications.[41] Care information miscommunication can happen at any time during the healthcare process, making it essential to teach and practice communication skills.

SIMULATION-BASED COMMUNICATION EXPERIENCES

MacLean and colleagues[15] noted communication failures as a leading cause of errors, yet communication continues to be a low priority in nursing education. After an SBE with video-reflective debriefing, learners reported having greater confidence in their communication and discharge teaching skills.[15] Teaching nurses to communicate with patients and families receiving palliative care or making decisions about end-of-life care is essential in all healthcare settings. Communicating the available resources and providing information that is understandable to the patient and family is a valuable communication skill.[28] Although the provider often relays bad news to patients, the nurse often answers questions after the patient and family has had time to process the information. Practicing palliative care and end-of-life scenarios through SBE and IPE has the potential to increase comfort in these situations and prepare healthcare teams to better dialogue with patients and families.[28]

SIMULATION STRATEGIES
Standardized Patients

Teaching communication skills requires interaction with others in real time. Use of SPs[42] can provide consistent, replicable learning experiences. Studies by Tian and colleagues[9] and Shao and colleagues[43] showed that integration of SPs in the role of parents and families had statistically significant impacts on communication skills and attitudes, including increased use of empathy and greater confidence in communication.

Virtual Reality

An additional strategy to teach communication is VR systems. Advances in VR allow for interactions with computer-based, virtual humans that are like face-to-face conversations.[1] These systems reinforce learning through repeated opportunities to speak, listen, assess, and respond to nonverbal actions. The use of virtual humans creates consistent experiences that can be replicated specific to the pedagogical design. Kron[1] and team used a VR system to train medical students advanced communication skills. The knowledge was retained and demonstrated in an Objective Structured Clinical Examination several days later.[1] Similarly, Choi and colleagues[44] used VR scenarios to teach communication skills by developing algorithmic videos for nursing students. Based on the virtual patient's response, the algorithm allowed learners to choose appropriate answers during scenario design. These answers were read and recorded as if they were responding to a live human, then played during the debrief. The team showed statistically significant differences in pretest and posttest results in learning self-efficacy and communication knowledge.[44] VR systems can have technological limitations that lead to frustration and less positive learning experiences, including discontent with speech recognition and poor replication of authentic clinical practices.[45,46]

Interprofessional Experiences

Simulation can be incorporated to learn interdisciplinary team communication, in low-stakes, psychologically safe environments.[6] TeamSTEPPS training and practice in the simulated environment potentially enhances learner comfort when speaking up within interprofessional teams to reduce the risk of hierarchical feelings of insecurity. Online communication training modules and VR have shown positive impacts on nurses' attitudes, knowledge, and skills when communicating.[29] Simulation serves as a valuable tool in communication education, providing learners with realistic and immersive experiences to enhance communication skills, teamwork, and patient-centered care for all health professionals.

Deliberate Practice

Teaching communication can also be accomplished through deliberate practice in simulation.[47] Deliberate practice is a technique used in SBE, implementing repetition to intentionally replace incorrect actions. In simulations that emphasized communication, Li[47] and colleagues used video recordings to assess the communication skills of nursing students. As part of the experimental process, learners critiqued their own videos and received feedback from their faculty twice per week for 8 weeks. The results showed a statistically significant difference in the learners' ability to establish rapport and respect, listen receptively, convey information effectively, and check perceptions when compared with learners who did not participate in the deliberate practice activities.[47]

Artificial Intelligence

Scenario development is an opportunity for nursing faculty to use ChatGPT (generative pretrained transformers) to assist in script writing. Chat GPT, a language model capable of generating communication simulations, makes it easier for faculty to develop scenario scripts.[48,49] The concern among academics is that this artificial intelligence chatbot makes it easier for learners to cheat; however, that is not usually an issue in SBE.[50] Although ChatGPT may not have a place in patient care in its current form, there is potential for artificial intelligence (AI) to enhance patient safety through critical alerts, scheduling and canceling of procedures due to discovered risks, and assisting with diagnosis, treatments, and cures of the future. Nursing faculty need to have the opportunity to learn and embrace AI to enhance communication teaching and learning.[48–50]

POST-COVID-19 COMMUNICATION

The COVID-19 pandemic provided evidence of the need to improve communication among healthcare systems. Misinformation about the virus, treatment, vaccinations, and patient safety was discussed internationally. However, positive innovations developed such as the increase in telehealth visits, recognition of the dwindling nursing workforce, need for improved stress management, and importance of better communication for safety of patients and caregivers.[51] A study by Simonovich and colleagues[51] reviewed communications of nurses during the beginning of the COVID-19 pandemic. They noted that effective communication positively affected nursing safety and patient outcomes.[51] Clear and concise communication by healthcare leaders and between nurses was essential for efficient operations. This required leaders' and nurses' presence, education, and emotional support to all members of the healthcare team.[51] Effective communication strategies during SBE, and translating those techniques into practice, will prepare the world and the nursing workforce for the future, ensuring that the catastrophic communication failures experienced during the COVID-19 pandemic remain in the past.[51]

SUMMARY

Effective communication is essential for improved patient outcomes. It is an essential part of global healthcare to ensure maintenance and support of the healthcare workforce. Teaching communication skills for nurse-patient-family education, team communication, conflict resolution and diversity, and equity is an opportunity for all health professionals to practice communication skills in a psychologically safe learning environment. This self-reflective learning strategy can uncover personal biases and how to manage them. This supports the vision of the healthcare workforce and industry becoming a place where all patients feel welcomed and comfortable sharing their healthcare needs and seeking treatment.

CLINICS CARE POINTS

- According to Janagama and colleagues,[2] and the NAM[3] in their landmark report, approximately 80% of all medical errors can be attributed to ineffective communication among healthcare teams and inadequate or confusing communication with patients and their families.
- Data show that $42 billion is spent on medication-related errors, and $12 billion of that loss can be attributed to ineffective communication.[2–5]
- Teaching and practicing effective communication skills has an impact on patient and family outcomes and improves patient care.

DISCLOSURE

The authors have nothing to disclose.

REFERENCES

1. Kron F, Fetters M, Scerbo M, et al. Using a computer simulation for teaching communication skills: A blinded multisite mixed methods randomized controlled trial. Patient Educ Counsel 2017;100(4):748–59.
2. Janagama S, Strehlow M, Gimkala A, et al. Critical communication: A cross-sectional study of sign out at the prehospital and Hospital interface. Cureus 2020;12(2). https://doi.org/10.7759/cureus.7114.

3. National Academies of Medicine. To err is human: Building a safer health system. National Academies Press; 1999. Available at: https://nap.nationalacademies. org/resource/9728/To-Err-is-Human-1999–report-brief.pdf.

4. Rodriguez-Perez J. An introduction to human errors. J Qual Participation 2019; 41(4). Available at: www.asq.org/pub/jqp.

5. Winterbottom F, Seoane L. Crossing the quality chasm: It takes a team to build the bridge. Ochsner J 2012;12(4):389–93.

6. Agency for Healthcare Research and Quality (AHRQ). Available at: https://www. ahrq.gov.

7. Hall K, Shoemaker-Hunt S, Hoffman L, Richard S, et al. Making healthcare safer III: a critical analysis of existing and emerging patient safety practices. (Prepared by Abt Associates Inc. under Contract No. 233-2015-00013-I.) AHRQ Publication No. 20-0029-EF. Rockville (MD): Agency for Healthcare Research and Quality; 2020. Available at: https://www.ahrq.gov/sites/default/files/wysiwyg/research/ findings/making-healthcare-safer/mhs3/making-healthcare-safer-III.pdf.

8. Tian J-D, Wu F-F, Wen C. Effects of teaching mode combining SimBaby with standardized patients on medical students' attitudes toward communication skills. BMC Med Educ 2022;22:825.

9. Wilkinson J, Treas L, Barnett K, et al. Fundamentals of nursing: Theory, concepts, and applications. Davis: F.A; 2020.

10. Richard E, Evans T, Williams B. Nursing students' perceptions of preparation to engage in patient education. Nurse Educ Pract 2018;28:1–6.

11. Diaz M, Dawson K. Impact of simulation-based closed loop communication training on medical errors in a pediatric emergency department. Am J Med Qual 2020;35(6):474–8.

12. Links M, Watterson L, Martin P, et al. Finding common ground: Meta-synthesis of communication frameworks found in patient communication, supervision and simulation literature. BMC Med Educ 2020;20:45–6.

13. Gutiérrez-Puertas L, Márquez-Hernández VV, Gutiérrez-Puertas V, et al. Educational interventions for nursing students to develop communication skills with patients: a systematic review. Int J Environ Res Publ Health 2020;17(7). https://doi. org/10.3390/ijerph17072241.

14. MacLean S, Kelly M, Geddes F, et al. Evaluating the use of teach-back in simulation training to improve discharge communication practices of undergraduate nursing students. Clinical Simulation in Nursing 2018;22:12–21.

15. Weiss EM, Piacentine BL, Candela L, et al. Effectiveness of using a simulation combined with online learning approach to develop discharge teaching skills. Nurse Educ Pract 2021;52. https://doi.org/10.1016/j.nepr.2021.103024.

16. Beaird G, Nye C, Thacker RL. The Use of Video Recording and Standardized Patient Feedback to Improve Communication Performance in Undergraduate Nursing Students. Clinical Simulation in Nursing 2017;13(4):176–85.

17. Markiewicz A, Hickman R, McAndrew N, et al. Enhancing palliative communication in the intensive care unit through simulation: A quality improvement project. Clinical Simulation in Nursing 2023;77:1–5.

18. Coleman D, McLaughlin D. Using simulated patients as a learning strategy to support undergraduate nurses to develop patient-teaching skills. Br J Nurs 2019;28(20):1300–6.

19. Griffiths B. Preparing tomorrow's nurses for collaborative quality care through simulation. Teach Learn Nurs 2018;13:46–60.

20. Lunde L, Moen A, Jakobsen R, et al. A preliminary simulation-based qualitative study of healthcare students' experiences of interprofessional primary care scenarios. Advances in Simulation 2022;7:1–12.

21. Mahmood L, Mohammed C, Gilbert J. Interprofessional simulation education to enhance teamwork and communication skills among medical and nursing undergraduates using the TeamSTEPPS® framework. Med J Armed Forces India 2021; 77(1):S42–8.

22. Foronda CL, Barroso S, Yeh VJ-H, et al. A rubric to measure nurse-to-physician communication: A pilot study. Clinical Simulation in Nursing 2021;50(C):38–42.

23. Kukko P, Silen-Lipponen M, Saaranen T. Health care students' perspectives about learning of affective interpersonal communication competence in interprofessional simulations. Nurse Educ Today 2020;94. https://doi.org/10.1016/j.nedt. 2020.104565.

24. Sowko AL, Fennimore AL, Drahnak MD. Teaching workplace Interprofessional Communication to undergraduate nursing students. J Nurs Educ 2019;58(9): 538–42.

25. Day L, Beard K. Meaningful inclusion of diverse voices: the case for culturally responsive teaching in nursing education. J Prof Nurs 2019;35:277–81.

26. Howard M, Embree J. Educational intervention improves communication abilities of nurses encountering workplace incivility. J Cont Educ Nurs 2020;51(3):138–44.

27. Van Gelderen S, Engebretson A, Miller A, et al. A family-care rubric: Developing family care and communication skills using simulation. Clinical Simulation in Nursing 2019;36:47–58.

28. Wittenberg E, Ferrell B, Kanter E, et al. Health literacy: Exploring nursing challenges to providing support and understanding. Clin J Oncol Nurs 2018;22: 53–61.

29. Chidume T. Teaching empathic communication at the end of life: a virtual simulation for nursing students. Nurs Educ Perspect 2022. https://doi.org/10.1097/01. NEP.0000000000001080.

30. Ottis E, Luetkenhaus K, Micheas L, et al. Assessing team communication with patients' families: Findings from utilizing the Communication Assessment Tool-Team (CAT-T) in an interprofessional error disclosure simulation. Patient Educ Counsel 2021;104:2292–6.

31. Chatman S, Wynn S. Improving healthcare access by teaching intercultural communication. J Christ Nurs 2021;38:52–6.

32. Boruff R. Preparing nursing students for enhanced communication with minority populations via simulation. Clinical Simulation in Nursing 2020;45:47–9.

33. Bonvicini K. LGBT healthcare disparities: What progress have we made? Patient Educ Counsel 2017;100:2357–61.

34. Cloyes K, Jones M, Gettens C, et al. Providing home hospice care for LGBTQ+ patients and caregivers: Perceptions and opinions of hospice interdisciplinary care team providers. Palliat Support Care 2023;21:3–11.

35. Ozdemir R, Erenoglu R. Attitudes of nursing students towards LGBT individuals and the affecting factors. Psychiatr Care 2022;58:239–47.

36. Turner J, Courtney R, Sarmiento E, et al. Frequency of safety net errors in the emergency department: Effect of patient handoffs. AJEM (Am J Emerg Med) 2021;42:188–91.

37. Bhattacharya K, Bhattacharya A, Bhattacharya N, et al, Published online February. ChatGPT in surgical practice: A new kid on the block. Indian J Surg 2023. https://doi.org/10.1007/s12262-023-03727-x.

38. Stevens Natalie, McNiesh S, Goyal D. Utilizing an SBAR Workshop With Baccalaureate Nursing Students to Improve Communication Skills". Nurs Educ Perspect 2020;41(2):117–8.
39. Raurell-Torredà Marta, Rascón-Hernán C, Malagón-Aguilera C, et al. Effectiveness of a training intervention to improve communication between/awareness of team roles: A randomized clinical trial". J Prof Nurs 2021;37(2):479–87.
40. Lee M, Lee S. Implementation of an electronic nursing record for nursing documentation and communication of patient care information in tertiary teaching hospital. Comput Inf Nurs 2021;39(3):136–44.
41. Lioce L, Lopreiato J, Founding Ed, Downing D, Chang TP, Robertson JM, Anderson M, Diaz DA, Spain AE, Terminology and concepts working group (2020). In: Healthcare simulation dictionary. 2nd edition. Rockville, MD: Agency for Healthcare Research and Quality; 2020. https://doi.org/10.23970/simulationv2. AHRQ Publication No. 20-0019.
42. Shao YN, Sun HM, Huang JW, et al. Simulation-based empathy training improves the communication skills of neonatal nurses. Clinical Simulation in Nursing 2018; 22:32–42.
43. Choi H, Lee U, Gwon T. Month). Development of a Computer Simulation-based, Interactive, Communication Education Program for Nursing Students. Clinical Simulation in Nursing 2021;56:1–9.
44. Shorey S, Ang E, Ng ED, et al. Communication skills training using virtual reality: A descriptive qualitative study. Nurse Educ Today 2020;94:104592.
45. Diaz DA, Shelton D, Anderson M, et al. The effect of simulation-based education on correctional health teamwork and communication. Clinical Simulation in Nursing 2019;27(C):1–11.
46. Li J, Li X, Gu L, et al. Effects of simulation-based deliberate practice on nursing students' communication, empathy, and self-efficacy. J Nurs Educ 2019;58(12): 681–9.
47. King K, Poor C, Gaudine A. Fostering Academic Success among English as an Additional Language Nursing Students Using Standardized Patients. Clinical Simulation in Nursing 2017;10:524–30.
48. Yardin E, Hutchinson M, Laycock R, et al. A chat (GPT) about the future of scientific publishing. Brain Behav Immun 2023;110:152–4.
49. Simonovich S, Spurlark R, Badowski D, et al. Examining effective communication in nursing practice during COVID-19: A large-scale qualitative study. Int Nurs Rev 2021;68:512–23.
50. Brink D. A nursing professor's response to chatGPT. International Journal of Nursing and Health Care Science 2023;03(02). Available at: https://columbuspublishers.com/uploads/articles/20230214112651223331_ijnhcs_2023_195.pdf.
51. Chen AS, Yau B, Revere L, et al. Implementation, evaluation, and outcome of TeamSTEPPS in interprofessional education: a scoping review. J Interprof Care 2019;33(6):795–804.

Breaking Barriers with Simulation-Enhanced Interprofessional Education
Transforming Interprofessional Education Through Simulation

Kelly Rossler, PhD, RN, CHSE, CNE[a],*,
Carman Turkelson, DNP, RN, CCRN-K, CHSE-A[b],
Jennifer Taylor, MSN, RN, NPD-BC, CCRN-K[c]

KEYWORDS

- Simulation • Interdisciplinary communication • Interprofessional collaboration
- Simulation standards • Nursing practice

KEY POINTS

- Nursing as a profession has prioritized interdisciplinary collaboration.
- Simulation-enhanced interprofessional education is a modality to teach collaborative practice skills.
- Interprofessional Education Collaborative Core Competencies and the Healthcare Simulation Standards of Best Practice: Sim-IPE are resources for learning interprofessional collaboration.

INTRODUCTION

As an iconic musical film, *My Fair Lady* highlights the impact of effective interprofessional communication and collaboration. In this musical, language coach, Professor Higgins, commences an endeavor to teach a flower seller described as having a lower-middle class dialect to speak English with such a flawless accent that the seller could be recognized as royalty.[1,2] Eliza Doolittle accepts the challenge and commences diction lessons to transform such lines as "The rain in spine sties minely in the pline" to the more eloquent "the rain in Spain stays mainly in the plain" to emerge

[a] Louise Herrington School of Nursing, Baylor University, 333 North Washington Avenue, Dallas, TX 75246, USA; [b] School of Nursing, University of Michigan-Flint, 303 East Kearsley Street, Flint, MI 48502, USA; [c] Baylor Scott & White Health Baylor University Medical Center, Center for Nursing Education and Research, 3500 Gaston Avenue, Dallas, TX 75246, USA
* Corresponding author.
E-mail address: Kelly_Rossler@baylor.edu

Nurs Clin N Am 59 (2024) 449–462
https://doi.org/10.1016/j.cnur.2024.01.007
0029-6465/24/© 2024 Elsevier Inc. All rights reserved.

as an articulate communicator. While this is a simplification of 1 storyline, throughout the musical, actors portrayed the roles of characters from diverse backgrounds and professions who develop a team dynamic that becomes central to the transformation of the lives of both student and coach. Less simplistic is the ever-evolving realm of healthcare delivery. It remains essential that foundational elements of interdisciplinary collaboration are maintained and sustained to meet the needs of the populations served. Simulation-enhanced interprofessional education (Sim-IPE) offers an avenue to teach and facilitate communication, collaboration, and teamwork while gaining an appreciation for the unique roles different healthcare professionals from a variety of settings bring to such learning experiences.[3] In nursing, interdisciplinary collaboration is not novel; however, the logistics of conducting Sim-IPE can become daunting as potential barriers emerge along the way. This article provides an initial overview of the current trajectory of interprofessional simulation-based education (SBE) in healthcare practice along with practical application within the varied workplaces where nurses are leaders within interdisciplinary teams seeking to speak the same language to deliver high-quality care.

Setting the Stage for Interprofessional Simulation-Based Education

While various nursing practice and licensure organizations and associations have informed the evolution of interprofessional SBE, a historical review of 2 invaluable resources, The Interprofessional Education Collaborative (IPEC) Core Competencies and the Healthcare Simulation Standards of Best Practice: Sim-IPE (HSSOBP™), is warranted.[3,4] Selected to provide context to this article, these 2 resources serve as a launching point for nurses seeking to learn more about Sim-IPE for integration into existing or future educational offerings. Since its original publication in 2011, the IPEC has continuously advocated for the healthcare industry to adopt interprofessional education (IPE) and collaborative practice (CP) to positively improve teamwork among health professionals which will in turn enhance healthcare outcomes.[5] Most recently, IPEC revealed the new 2023 Core Competencies designed to "empower the IPE community with the best available evidence and research" on both IPE and CP.[3,6] While influences from research have informed policy and subsequent changes to practice behaviors, the new Core Competencies offer nurses 4 key tenets and 33 associated competency statements encompassing (a) values and ethics, (b) roles and responsibilities, (c) communication, and (d) teams and teamwork.[3,6] The new competency statements also reflect changes to nursing education standards focused on competency-based education offered by the American Association of Colleges of Nursing in the *Essentials* and Research Priorities of the National Institute of Nursing Research.[7,8] On the acute care side, the Forces of Magnetism model envisioned by the American Nurses Credentialing Center for the Magnet Recognition Program offers nurses practicing in hospital settings a pathway to attain excellence within realms of practice and research as a member of an interprofessional team addressing global healthcare and nursing issues.[9] Similarly, nursing practice organizations/associations from academia, community and public health, and rural health, to school nursing have identified priorities associated with interdisciplinary collaboration as essential[10–13] Finally, IPE and CP are crucial to military nurses and nurse leaders serving in the armed forces during times of peace and when preparing to deliver combat casualty care (**Fig. 1**).[14,15]

Identified as a priority in the early 2010s, the Sim-IPE standard joined a compendium of existing standards representing best practices of simulation pedagogy in 2015 and was most recently revised with the HSSOBP™ in 2021.[4] Serving as aspirational guidelines for simulationists trained to facilitate interprofessional SBEs, this standard consists of 4 criteria necessary to teach IPE and CP using simulation-based teaching

School Nursing	Community & Public Health Nursing	Rural Nursing	Military Nursing
• Preparedness & Response: Disasters & Emergencies • School Well-Being • Health Equity and Social Determinants of Health • Coordination of Care: Acute & Chronic Conditions	• Collaboration • Advocacy • Leadership • Mentorship • Equity in the Workforce	• Diversity in Rural Practice • Quality Education and Healthcare in Communities • Interprofessional Education	• Trauma Care • Research and Development • Civilian Partnerships • Mission Readiness

Fig. 1. Practice priorities in diverse nursing roles.

modalities. The criteria encompass (a) the use of a theoretic or conceptual framework to conduct Sim-IPE, (b) the use of best practices to design and develop Sim-IPE, (c) recognizing and addressing potential obstacles, and (d) developing a plan to evaluate Sim-IPE. Fortunately, literature on research and evidence-based practice protocols from across the globe provide insight as to the status of Sim-IPE to support nurse educators and simulationists seeking to conduct Sim-IPE in the context of their current practice environment while placing due consideration on future areas for consideration such as impact on patient care outcomes and as a potential return on investment post implementation.[16–25] A word cloud representation was created from literature spanning a 5-year timeframe as to the overarching focus areas for SBE within nursing practice settings (**Fig. 2**).[16–25]

Creating Simulation-Enhanced Interprofessional Education Experiences

Once again, the IPEC Core Competencies and HSSOBP[TM] Sim-IPE provide insight and a framework for designing, implementing, and evaluating unique Sim-IPE experiences.[3,4] In the following paragraphs, the authors provide guidance along with examples on how to create Sim-IPE experiences unique to your practice environment and needs. The 2 exemplars offer a review of pre-development considerations to be mindful of when designing Sim-IPE experiences using the HSSOBP[TM] Sim-IPE within your organization.[3,4] The first exemplar travels through the development of a Sexual Assault Nurse Examiner (SANE) courtroom experience for a university-based SANE certification program.[26] The second exemplar offers a glimpse of a community-based mass casualty Sim-IPE event encompassing multiple agencies across a rural community (**Boxes 1–4**).

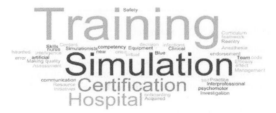

Fig. 2. Simulation-enhanced interprofessional education use in practice.

Think about location, models, and frameworks

Although Sim-IPE may traditionally take place within an academic setting, many Sim-IPE activities are well suited for locations within the community or acute care settings. Regardless of the setting, it will be important to consider a theoretic model or conceptual framework that will serve to guide the development and implementation of the Sim-IPE. There are several adult learning theories that could be utilized along with the IPEC Core Competencies and IPE training as well as the model conceptualization process that could be considered for your institution[4,27–29] (**Fig. 3**).

Stakeholders and keeping an eye on potential challenges

Identfying key stakeholders is a crucial first step in sucessfully planning for Sim-IPE. Without buy-in from key stakeholders as well as the completion of a needs assessment validating the need and focus for the Sim-IPE, implementation barriers may be encountered.[3,4] (see **Box 1**).

Successful planning and development of a Sim-IPE requires consultation and collaboration with experts as well as representatives of the targeted interprofessional learners. The planning phases should include discussions around mutual goals and objectives for the learners as well as identification of realistic activities or scenarios to support attainment of the goals and objectives identified. It is important to remember that establishment of mutual goals and objectives across multiple professions requires communication and collaboration among the experts.[3,4] During these discussions, keep an eye on the goals of Sim-IPE which focus on interprofessional competencies versus professional knowledge, skills, and attitudes. During this phase, it will be equally important to identify potential barriers or challenges with implementation early! This will enable the team to address any potential barriers before they occur and will help facilitate the implementation of the Sim-IPE. *EXPERT TIP: Planning Sim-IPE often takes additional time and planning to coordinate multiple professions whether within the acute care setting or community. Be sure to allocate adequate time for this! There are also unique challenges and barriers to Sim-IPEs such as time, space, financial resources, and long-term sustainability.

Design and development

The design and development of a Sim-IPE should follow best practices in simulation design and begin with defining learning objectives that focus on interprofessional competencies and collaboration.[3,4] Other key considerations include identification of the roles of the different healthcare or other professionals involved and deciding on the scenarios or patient cases to be used. One challenge at this stage may encompass aligning objectives with the standards of practice for the multiple professions involved in the Sim-IPE. Additionally, the scenarios or patient cases must be carefully designed in a way that fosters collaboration and interaction among the different professionals. Each professional should have an active role in the scenario or patient care

---

Box 1
Identification of stakeholders: A SANE exemplar

Key stakeholders include expert and novice SANEs, Sexual Assault and Child Advocacy Centers, prosecutors, judges, victims' advocates, and law enforcement, subject matter experts, simulationists, and simulation operationalists. Prior to development of this Sim-IPE, key stakeholders were contacted. During the discussions with key stake holders, all identified an interest in participating in a mock court room Sim-IPE as well as a need for additional training and education around SANE testimony at a trial.

Box 2
Unique challenges to the sexual assault nurse examiner simulation-enhanced interprofessional education

Time: The planning and development of an 8-h immersive Sim-IPE SANE mock court room experience took 6 months with multiple meetings via video conferencing to identify profession-specific goals and objectives. Coming to consensus on goals centered around the Sim-IPE experience was crucial to success.

Realism: The identification of multiple sexual assault (SA) cases that were criminally prosecuted was discussed as potential options for the development of 2 different simulated mock court cases. Using real cases as a framework for the Sim-IPE scenario design created realism and provided learners with multiple opportunities to engage with other professionals (judges, prosecutors, and defense attorneys) while serving in the role of the SANE expert providing during the testimony phase of the simulation. Having this event occur in an actual courthouse further enhanced realism. However, this necessitated the event to take place on a weekend when the court was not in use.

Logistics: Navigation of complex schedules of expert professionals to ensure the Sim-IPE did not infringe on daily role responsibilities within their respective communities. Being mindful of the practice schedules of participating nurses was also paramount. Scheduling 8 weeks in advance of the event allowed the team to navigate potential scheduling barriers. Having a dedicated person to coordinate delivery of necessary educational materials, manage attendance tracking, keep time, organize lunch, and ensure completion of surveys was crucial to success.

Resources: Integrating resources such as the IPEC and HSSOBP™ guidelines to ensure core IPE concepts are represented was a critical consideration. In addition to the SANE subject matter expert used to develop this Sim-IPE, multiple resources primarily from community partners were required for successfull implementation. Given that the event was held in the community, the simulation team had to provide support at an off-site location. Another consideration involved exploring if there was a need for financial support to conduct the Sim-IPE (eg, payment for experts, food, and other resources/supplies).

---

based on their profession's standards and scope of practice. The design and development of a Sim-IPE scenario must also integrate the expertise representatives from the multiple professions who will be partaking in the experience. Failure to do so may result in decreased realism, buy-in, and inability of learners to fully engage in the Sim-IPE experience[4] (**Boxes 2–4**).

Pre-learning/Pre-briefing

Prior to the Sim-IPE, a pre-briefing session should be held to inform participants about the goals and expectations of the simulation, the roles they are expected to play, the simulation environment, and the equipment to be used. In the setting of a Sim-IPE, the pre-brief should also encompass team-based concepts and pre-learning activities that will support the goals and objectives of the Sim-IPE.[4,30] It is imperative that all learners have access to the team-based knowledge and information to successfully engage in the Sim-IPE and achieve the desired learning objectives.[3] This often requires the learner to have access to pre-learning activities (readings, lectures, videos, or other content), expectations, and the goals and objectives of the simulation experience prior to the actual day of the Sim-IPE.[27,30] This can be done in a variety of ways including pre-learning materials and activities posted on-line in a learning management system for asynchronous learning and review pre-simulation, and/or in-person through a discussion with simulation faculty immediately prior to the Sim-IPE.

There are several options for interprofessional team-based training. One team-based curricular resource utilized by nursing and healthcare teams is Team- STEPPS.[31]

Box 3
Unique challenges to large-scale disaster simulation-enhanced interprofessional education

Time: Planning and development of an 8-h large full-scale community-based disaster Sim-IPE with representatives from the local fire departments, local and state police, public safety, rural and community hospitals, emergency medical response teams (EMS), 9-1-1 or community central dispatch, medical flight teams, health department Red Cross, the university, and the mock exercise site required a full year to plan. Meetings took place in person at the emergency management center for the community where the different professions worked through development of the goals and objectives as well as identification of individual sub-objectives for their teams.

Realism: Volunteer nursing students and community members served as injured participants. Moulage and other make-up were used to mimic injuries. Each volunteer was provided que cards to indicate key specifics such as vital signs and other details. Supplies required from the simulation center also included pre-made wounds along with simulation center staff to assist with application of moulage.

Logistics: Logistics went beyond identification of a site to include 1) identification of coverage for all of the professions and sites involved to ensure that public and patient safety was not compromised during the mock disaster exercise, 2) clear communication plan for the community prior to and the day of the exercise to ensure public safety and prevent miscommunication, 3) identification of the radio communication channel for the mock exercise separate from the standard radio communication channels for actual events to prevent confusion, 4) pre-learning activities for the site (eg, high-school, courtroom, church, senior center) and all participants, 5) as this was an 8-hour event, access to water, bathrooms, and food were also important logistics to consider. Donations were sought from community agencies to provide coffee, hot-cocoa, bathrooms, and lunch during the debriefing, 6) expecting the unexpected, consideration also had to be given for inclement weather during the events that were scheduled to be outdoors.

This patient-focused curriculum offered by the Agency for Healthcare Research and Quality was revised in 2023 to speak to current interprofessional educational modalities offered to nurses and healthcare teams to optimize preparedness for practice in the ever-changing healthcare practice environment. From implementation guides to

---

Box 4
Questions to explore

Exploring the location of the Sim-IPE is necessary to ensure there is adequate space and resources to accommodate the Sim-IPE. Ask these questions and more!

Is the event is taking place outside of a traditional simulation center, where will this be?

Do you need to have approval to use the off-site location? What is the process? How long might this take?

Will it require the site/location to stop usual operations, or will the event need to take place on a weekend or at a time when the location is not operating?

What resources are necessary to operationalize the Sim-IPE off site?

Does the event require transportation of equipment and simulation staff to support the event?

How many participants are expected? How many facilitators are needed? What professions will be represented? How will all professions be engaged in the Sim-IPE?

What equipment or supplies will be needed to facilitate the Sim-IPE?

Is there access to water, bathrooms, food? Will lunch/water need to be provided?

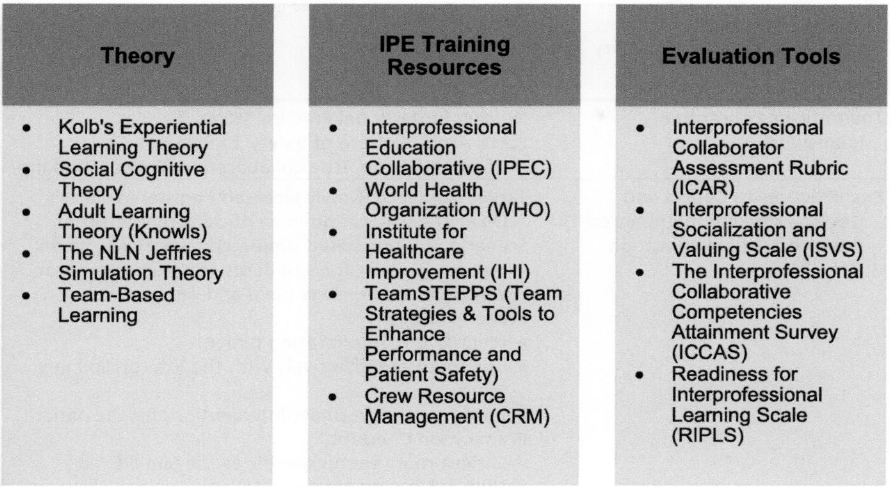

Theory	IPE Training Resources	Evaluation Tools
• Kolb's Experiential Learning Theory • Social Cognitive Theory • Adult Learning Theory (Knowls) • The NLN Jeffries Simulation Theory • Team-Based Learning	• Interprofessional Education Collaborative (IPEC) • World Health Organization (WHO) • Institute for Healthcare Improvement (IHI) • TeamSTEPPS (Team Strategies & Tools to Enhance Performance and Patient Safety) • Crew Resource Management (CRM)	• Interprofessional Collaborator Assessment Rubric (ICAR) • Interprofessional Socialization and Valuing Scale (ISVS) • The Interprofessional Collaborative Competencies Attainment Survey (ICCAS) • Readiness for Interprofessional Learning Scale (RIPLS)

Fig. 3. Theory, resources, and evaluation tools.

simulation videos and key concepts of team dynamics, this robust curriculum can be self-paced or adopted as an organizational training program. **Fig. 3** also presents team building resources for potential adoption within your Sim-IPE program.[4,31–33]

Conducting the Simulation
The Sim-IPE should be facilitated by trained simulation faculty with knowledge and expertise within the realm of simulation pedagogy.[4] The method of facilitation should reflect the goals of the Sim-IPE and provide learners from multiple professions with demonstration and practice of their interprofessional collaborative competencies. Additional training may be needed for facilitators of Sim-IPE around best practices of simulation; therefore, it is important to consider this in the initial planning.

Debriefing
Immediately after the Sim-IPE, an interprofessional debriefing session should be held. As with any simulation, the goal of the interprofessional debriefing session is to foster learner reflection and learning from successes and mistakes.[4,34,35] Debriefing is also essential to allow for clarification, deep learning, meaning making, and transference. However, it is important to recognize that a Sim-IPE debriefing is different from a traditional debriefing in that it should include representatives of the different professions participating and led by trained simulation faculty to discuss the simulations' events, outcomes, and participants' experiences.[3,4,34,35] Having facilitators for a Sim-IPE who represent the multiple professions helps provide the role-specific context during the debriefing, which is important to the interprofessional learners.

Using an interprofessional/team-based debriefing model or format that aligns with your organization can help facilitate an interprofessional debriefing approach.[4] This aspect may also require some additional training and discussion among the interprofessional team facilitating the simulation prior to the actual Sim-IPE. One approach to ensure all professions are represented is described as a co-debriefing process.[36] Using this approach, 2 or more persons facilitate the Sim-IPE debriefing with the added focus on gaining perspectives from among the learners to gain a better understanding of practice-specific roles within the team. Another potential option for an interprofessional Sim-IPE debriefing is to use a 2-tiered approach where 2 distinct debriefings are

Table 1
Hospital-based nurse residency and internship experience

HSSOBP™ Sim-IPE Criteria	Exemplar
Theoretic or Conceptual Framework	Nursing Professional Practice Model[29] Focus Areas: Culture of Safety, Effective Communication, True Collaboration, Critical Thinking
Best Practices to Design and Develop simulation-enhanced interprofessional education (Sim-IPE)	Target Audience: Newly Licensed Registered Nurses (NLRNs) participating in a critical care internship. Scenario: Pre-purchased simulated scenarios from an industry partner for 3 patients admitted for motor vehicle accident, chest pain, and sepsis. Scenario Objectives: • Identify the deteriorating patient. • Communicate effectively with the interdisciplinary team. • Implement appropriate interventions for the patient. Preparation Checklist: • Patient room set up specific to the Sim-IPE. • High-fidelity mannequin • Relevant equipment (current), demonstration only medications (labeled), single use supplies, mock patient cart with orders, and nursing documentation. • Verify debriefing location (same as Sim-IPE). Debriefing: • Verify debriefing model and training of facilitator for selected debriefing model. • Explore pre-purchased simulated scenarios for Sim-IPE-specific debriefing.
Recognize and Address Potential Obstacles	• Number of NLRNs in the same internship cohort • Facilitator: Voice of the patient and/or provider • Sim-IPE is in alignment with the NLRN's preceptor schedule
Evaluation of Sim-IPE	• Internal Exit to Practice Evaluation Tool • Creighton Competency Evaluation Instrument [Complete inter-rater reliability]

Adapted from the Healthcare Simulation Standards of Best Practice: Sim-IPE (HSSOBP™).[4]

held.[4,37,38] With this debriefing approach, the intent is to conduct an initial debriefing after the Sim-IPE that focuses solely on the patient care objectives that are unique to each profession. The second debriefing would then be focused solely on interprofessional team dynamics and teamwork objectives.[37]

Evaluation and program assessment

Identification of valid and reliable IPE-focused tools to assess the achievement of the goals and objectives and/or performance of the learners is another consideration in this process.[3,4] Again, it will be important to consider the HSSOBP™ and utilize evaluation tools and learner assessments that align with Sim-IPE learning objectives and focus on measuring the learners' ability to work effectively, communicate, collaborate, and work within an interprofessional team.[3,4] Finally, after the Sim-IPE, consider soliciting additional feedback and encourage self-reflection within the Sim-IPE development team to ensure continuous improvement and learning.[4,31,32] Each time a Sim-IPE is conducted, valuable insight is gained allowing for modification or fine-tuning of the Sim-IPE activities based on feedback and assessment results.[35,39–41]

Putting it all together
When seeking to integrate the components of Sim-IPE into your organizational struc-ture, snippets from how interprofessional education and collaboration were included in a well-established critical care nursing internship offered by a university medical center are shared (**Table 1**). Additionally, a safety room assessment focused on hospital-acquired pressure injury for training of healthcare teams is provided (**Table 2**). When conceptualizing the development of Sim-IPE, writing down initial ideas that become final products is highly encouraged. Additionally, using an estab-lished template such as the National League for Nursing simulation design template offers a means to customize the learning experience while maintaining high-quality simulation.[40] For this exemplar, the HSSOPB™: Sim-IPE criteria are used to illustrate use of the guidelines. [4] Additionally, a scenario involving a patient emergency man-agement experience allows for interdisciplinary teams serving in diverse levels of care areas to develop and execute communication and collaboration skills (**Table 3**). For such an exemplar, readily available resources from the American Heart Association, The Joint Commission, National Institute of Health (NIH) Stroke Scale,

Table 2
Safety room assessment: hospital-acquired pressure injury

Objectives:
• Identify conditions that increase the patient's risk for hospital-acquired pressure injury (HAPI).
• Discuss interventions to prevent such issues.

Facilitator Guide	
Instructions to Learners	• You will have 15 min to assess the room and identify safety concerns.
	• You should enter and leave the room just as you would for a real patient.
	• Assess the patient and the room just like you would a real patient.
	• Write safety concerns identified on paper provided.
	• When you are finished with your assessment, exit the room and wait in the hallway.
	• When everyone has completed their assessment, we will discuss the safety concerns noted as a group.
	• Complete the roster after the scheduled debriefing
Debriefing 15–30 min	• Co-Debriefing with Facilitators
	• Utilize whiteboard in the room for debriefing.
	• Start with "Will someone tell me what they think is one of the biggest patient safety risks in this room"?
	• Discussion among participants: At risk behaviors, corrective actions, policies to follow, identify un-recognized safety risks.
Safety Risks	
Bedding	• Multiple layers of bedding under the patient
	• Wrinkles/bunching of linen under patient
	• Fitted sheet over waffle
Devices	• Waffle over-inflated; under fitted sheet
	• Patient laying on foley tubing with clamp under thigh
	• Ventilator tubing placing pressure on patient's lip.
	• Nasogastric tube not bridled; taped directly against nares.
Patient	• Improper incontinence care
	• Foam dressing not applied appropriately
	• Patient is supine
	• Braden Score total is incorrect
	• Heels not floated- either pillow or foam boot

Table 3
Stroke management exemplar

Scenario: Stroke Management	
Design Considerations	
Setting	Ambulance Bay, Emergency Department, computed tomography (CT) Scanner
Target Audience	Team Trained in Stroke Management (Initial or Ongoing Validation)
Participants	Emergency medical response teams (EMS) personnel, Pharmacist, Emergency Department staff, Respiratory Therapy, CT Technicians, Family members. Patient actor for NIH assessment (Standardized Patient)
Supplies	Relevant equipment (current), practice medications, single use supplies for each simulation group. Mock patient chart, orders, facility-relevant policies/guidelines, and nurse documentation template. • Simulation medications: alteplase, normal saline flushes, aspirin, nicardipine infusion, intravenous (IV) push anti-hypertensives, medications for ventilator management, IV fluids. • Simulation mannequin(s) that allow airway management, peripheral intravenous catheter access, central lines, indwelling urinary catheters, and hemodynamic monitoring. • Single use supplies including: IV start kits, intubation tray, arterial line insertion and monitoring kit, suction equipment etc.
Resources	• American Heart Association (AHA) Adult Suspected Stroke Algorithm[42,43] • The Joint Commission Standardized Performance Measures for Comprehensive Stroke Centers.[44] • National Institute of Health (NIH) Stroke Scale.[45] • Hospital-specific order sets, guidelines, protocols for stroke activation and management

Scenario Script		
Scenario	Critical Steps	MET

EMS contacts emergency department with stroke activation for patient in route. Patient enters emergency department via EMS accompanied by family.
• Patient is a 78-year-old male.
• Last known well time is 2 h ago.
• Vital Signs on arrival:
  ○ Blood Pressure: 176/90
  ○ Heart Rate: 55- Sinus bradycardia
  ○ SPO$_2$: 94
  ○ Resp: 18
• Past medical history: Type 2 DM, Hyperlipidemia, Chronic obstructive pulmonary disease- current smoker
• Medications: Metformin, Crestor, Baby Aspirin, Symbicort.
• No known drug allergy
• Blood glucose: 250
• NIH Stroke Scale: 8
	Activate Stroke Team
	Prepare for emergent computed tomography (CT)
	Measure vital signs, place patient on monitor, administer oxygen if needed. Assess for airway protection.
	If stable, immediately to CT scan.
	Obtain IV access
	Obtain point of care blood glucose
	Interview family/patient for past medical history, medications, and allergies
	Determine symptom onset- last known well time
	Assess patient and perform NIH Stroke Scale Assessment
	Review brain imaging for intercranial hemorrhage
	Assess for alteplase eligibility—inclusion criteria and absolute contraindications. (Checklist)	

(continued on next page)

Table 3 (*continued*)		
Scenario Script		
Scenario	**Critical Steps**	**MET**
• CT scan: No evidence of intracranial hemorrhage • Alteplase administration	Administer alteplase—Reconstitution of medication per manufacture instructions for use, calculation of dose, and correct programming of IV pump. Monitor and treat arterial hypertension Evaluate for endovascular therapy Transfer to higher level of care	

Eligibility Recommendations for IV Alteplase in Adult Patients with Acute Ischemic Stroke – Indications

☐ Acute ischemic stroke symptoms

☐ Symptoms onset within 4.5 hours

☐ CT head without intracranial hemorrhage

☐ BP > 185/110 mm Hg at time of tPA infusion (BP reduction to goal with two agents recommended with physician assessing the stability of the BP before starting IV alteplase)

Absolute Contraindications (**NONE** of the boxes should be checked)

☐ Evidence of acute intracranial hemorrhage on pretreatment evaluation

☐ Symptoms determined to be Mild AND Nondisabling

☐ CT brain imaging exhibits severe/extensive regions of clear hypoattenuation/frank hypodensity

☐ Previous ischemic stroke within the prior 3 months as determined by physician

☐ Presence of severe head trauma, whether acute or recent within the prior 3 months as determined by physician

☐ Intracranial or intraspinal surgery within prior 3 months

☐ History of intracranial hemorrhage

☐ High clinical suspicion of subarachnoid hemorrhage

☐ Known intracranial AND intra-axial neoplasm

☐ Clinical symptoms suggesting infective endocarditis

☐ Known or suspected aortic arch dissection

☐ GI malignancy

☐ Active internal bleeding including GI bleed within 21 days as determined by physician

☐ Presence of a bleeding diathesis or coagulopathy as defined by

  o Platelets < 100,000/mm3 (In patients without history of thrombocytopenia, treatment with IV alteplase can be initiated before availability of platelet count but should be discontinued if platelet count is <100,000/mm3)

  o INR > 1.7 (In patients without recent use of OACs or heparin, treatment with IV alteplase can be initiated before availability of coagulation test results but should be discontinued if INR >1.7)

  o aPTT > 40 secs

  o PT > 15 secs (In patients without recent use of OACs or heparin, treatment with IV alteplase can be initiated before availability of coagulation test results but should be discontinued with elevated PT)

☐ Full treatment dose LMWH within previous 24 hours

☐ Concurrent use of Glycoprotein IIb/IIIa receptor inhibitors[a]

☐ Concurrent use of direct thrombin inhibitors[b] or direct factor Xa inhibitors[b] and at least one of the following criteria:

  o Appropriate laboratory tests (aPTT, INR, ecarin clotting time, thrombin time, or direct factor Xa activity assays) are abnormal

  o Patient has taken a dose of the above in the last 48 hours

[a] Glycoprotein IIb/IIIa receptor inhibitors: Abciximab (Reopro), Eptifibatide (Integrilin), Tirofiban (Aggrastat) [b] Oral factor Xa and direct thrombin inhibitors: Apixaban (Eliquis), Betrixaban (Bevyxxa), Edoxaban (Savaysa), Rivaroxaban (Xarelto), and Dabigatran (Pradaxa)

Physician Signature: Provider#   Date: Time:

Last updated 02/2020; Adapted from 2019 AHA/ASA Guideline for the Early Management of Patients With Acute Ischemic Stroke: 2019 Update. Powers, WJ.

Abbreviations: MET, completed critical step.

and internal policy documents supported the development and implementation of this Sim-IPE.[42–45]

SUMMARY

Throughout one's professional education and growth in nursing, diverse and impactful experiences can culminate into a rewarding career informed during interactions as a member of an interdisciplinary team. As SBE continues to be infused within practice settings, more opportunities exist to transform not only individual practice behaviors but also the institutions in which nurses practice; hopefully culminating in how interdisciplinary teams positively impact healthcare outcomes. When seeking to cultivate an environment where Sim-IPE is prevalent, using and adapting readily available resources offers multiple benefits to both learners and institutions. Commencing your first Sim-IPE experience can be a pivotal step in developing a sustainable program that will grow to fit the evolving needs of those nurses interact with and perform alongside every day.

CLINICS CARE POINTS

- Nursing practice associations and organizations from across all nursing practice sectors have identified priorities focused on interdisciplinary collaboration.

- SIM-IPE offers an avenue to teach and facilitate communication, collaboration, and teamwork among healthcare professionals.

- The Interprofessional Education Collaborative Core Competencies and the Healthcare Simulation Standards of Best Practice: Sim-IPE are resources for learning of interprofessional collaborative practice behaviors.

DISCLOSURE

Authors have no disclosures to report.

REFERENCES

1. Margolies D. "My Fair Lady at the Ahmanson Theatre." Back Stage West, vol. 15, no. 16, 2008, p. 18. Gale OneFile: Fine Arts, link.gale.com/apps/doc/A178897070/PPFA?u=txshracd2488&sid=bookmark- PPFA&xid=5cb1d048. Accessed 14 Nov. 2023.
2. Lerner AJ, My Fair Lady Loewe C. Video. Warner Bros. Pictures; 1998.
3. Interprofessional Education Collaborative. Core competencies for interprofessional collaborative practice: Preliminary draft revisions. 2023. Available at: https://www.ipecollaborative.org/ipec-core-competencies. [Accessed 2 July 2023].
4. INACSL Standards Committee, Rossler K, Molloy M, Pastva A, et al. Healthcare simulation standards of best practice™ simulation-enhanced interprofessional education. Clin Simul Nurs 2021 Sept;58:49–53.
5. Interprofessional Education Collaborative. IPEC announces working group members for core competencies revision update of IPEC core competencies to begin June 2021. Available at: https://www.ipecollaborative.org/assets/press-release/IPEC_Press-Release_2021-05-04_CCR-WG-Announcement.pdf. [Accessed 2 July 2023].
6. Interprofessional Education Collaborative. Core competencies for interprofessional collaborative practice: version 3. Washington, DC: Interprofessional Education Collaborative. Available at: https://www.ipecollaborative.org/assets/core-competencies/IPEC_Core_Competencies_Version_3_2023.pdf. [Accessed 7 January 2024].
7. American Association of Colleges of Nursing. The Essentials: Core competencies for professional nursing education. 2021. Available at: https://www.aacnnursing.org/Portals/0/PDFs/Publications/Essentials-2021.pdf. [Accessed 15 July 2023].
8. National Institute of Nursing Research. The National Institute of Nursing Research 2022-2026 Strategic Plan. Available at: https://www.ninr.nih.gov/aboutninr/ninr-mission-and-strategic-plan. [Accessed 15 July 2023].
9. American Nurses Credentialing Center. AACN Magnet Recognition Program. Available at: https://www.nursingworld.org/organizational-programs/magnet/. [Accessed 15 July 2023].
10. National Association of School Nurses. The National Association of School Nurses Research and Research Implementation Priorities 2023. Available at: https://www.nasn.org/research/research-priorities. [Accessed 15 July 2023].

11. Association of Community Health Nursing Educators. Research & Evidence-Based Practice Project Priorities. 2020. Available at: https://www.nasn.org/research/research-priorities. [Accessed 15 July 2023].

12. Nurse Organization Rural. International Rural Nursing Conference. 2023. Available at: https://www.rno.org/2023-IRNC-Conference. [Accessed 1 September 2023].

13. National Council of State Boards of Nursing. NCSBN's environmental scan: nursing at a crossroads – an opportunity for action. Available at: J. Nurs Regul Epub 2023;13(Supplement):S1–48 www.journalofnursingregulation.com.

14. Ma H, Chihava TN, Fu J, et al. Competencies of military nurse managers: A scoping review and unifying framework. J Nurs Manag 2020;28(6):1166–76.

15. Hefley J, Talbot LA, Metter EJ, et al. Advancing readiness through military programs: An evidence-based practice perspective. Mil Med 2023;189(Supplement_1):31–8.

16. Jang EC. Addressing challenges to the development, delivery, and evaluation of continuing education for nurses. Nurs Clin North Am 2022;57(4):513–23.

17. Kaminski-Ozturk N, Martin B. Virtual clinical simulation adoption and use by licensed practical nurse/licensed vocational nurse education programs during the COVID-19 pandemic. J Nurs Regul 2023;14(1):21–9.

18. Toft LEB, Bottinor W, Cobourn A, et al. A simulation-enhanced, spaced learning, interprofessional "code blue" curriculum improves ACLS algorithm adherence and trainee resuscitation skill confidence. J Interprof Care 2023;37(4):623–8.

19. Gilbert M, Waxman KT, Gilbert GE, et al. The scope of hospital-based simulation. J Nurs Adm 2021;51(2):74–80.

20. Saraswathy T, Nalliah S, Rosliza AM, et al. Applying interprofessional simulation to improve knowledge, attitude and practice in hospital- acquired infection control among health professionals. BMC Med Educ 2021;21(1):482–91.

21. Vaughn J, Blodgett NP, Molloy MA. Haunted hospital: an innovative and engaging approach to interprofessional education simulation. J Interprof Educ Pract 2023; 32:100645.

22. Cant R, Cooper SJ, Lam LL. Hospital nurses' simulation-based education regarding patient safety: a scoping review. Clin Simul Nurs 2020;44:19–34.

23. Rutherford-Hemming T, Alfes CM. The use of hospital-based simulation in nursing education – a systematic review. Clin Simul Nurs 2017;13:78–89.

24. Abualenain J. Hospital-wide interprofessional simulation-based training in crisis resource management. Eurasian J Med 2018;17(3):93–6. https://doi.org/10.5152/eajem.2018.49389.

25. Rossler KL, Hardin K, Taylor J. Teaching interprofessional socialization and collaboration to nurses transitioning into critical care. Clin Simul Nurs 2020;49:9–15.

26. Dickinson KJ, Ward WL, Minarcin R, et al. An interprofessional medical malpractice mock trial: event evolution and assessment of efficacy. Int J Healthc Simul 2023;1–12. https://doi.org/10.54531/zxmk6987.

27. Jeffries PR. The NLN Jeffries simulation theory. 2nd edition. Wolters Kluwer: National League for Nursing; 2021.

28. Gilbert JH, Yan J, Hoffman SJ. A WHO report: framework for action on interprofessional education and collaborative practice. J Allied Health 2010;39(Suppl 1):196–7. PMID: 21174039.

29. Bradley D, Dixon JF. Staff nurses creating safe passage with evidence-based practice. Nurs Clin N Am 2009;44:71–81. https://doi.org/10.1016/j.cnur.2008.10.002.

30. INACSL Standards Committee, McDermott DS, Ludlow J, Horsley E, et al. Healthcare Simulation Standards of Best Practice™ Prebriefing: Preparation and Briefing. Clin Simul Nurs 2021;58:9–13. September).

31. Agency for Healthcare Research and Quality. TeamSTEPPS. Available at: https://www.ahrq.gov/teamstepps-program/index.html. [Accessed 15 September 2023].
32. Institute for Healthcare Improvement. Career growth and professional development. 2023. Available at: https://www.ihi.org/education. [Accessed 1 November 2023].
33. Buljac-Samardžić M, Dekker-van Doorn CM, Maynard MT. What do we really know about crew resource management in healthcare?: an umbrella review on crew resource management and its effectiveness. J Patient Saf 2021;17(8): e929–58.
34. INACSL Standards Committee, Decker S, Alinier G, Crawford SB, et al. Healthcare Simulation Standards of Best PracticeTM The Debriefing Process. Clinical Simulation in Nursing 2021;58:27–32.
35. Smith L, Keiser M, Yorke A, et al. Use of a structured approach to develop best practices in interprofessional education. J Nurs Educ 2021;60(6):309–16.
36. Goldsworthy S, Goodhand K, Baron S, et al. Co-debriefing Virtual Simulations: An International Perspective. Clin Simul Nurs 2022;63:1–4.
37. Andersen P, Coverdale S, Kelly M, et al. Interprofessional simulation: developing teamwork using a two-tiered debriefing approach. Clin Simul Nurs 2018;20:15–23.
38. Shrader S, Farland MZ, Danielson J, et al. A systematic review of assessment tools measuring interprofessional education outcomes relevant to pharmacy education. Am J Pharmaceut Educ 2017;81(6):119.
39. Nexus Resource Exchange. Collection of existing interprofessional practice and education measurement instruments. National Center for Interprofessional Practice and Education. Available at: https://nexusipe.org/advancing/assessment-evaluation. [Accessed 1 October 2023].
40. National League for Nursing. Simulation design template. Originally adapted from Childs, Sepples, Chambers. Designing simulations for nursing education. In: Jeffries PR, editor. Simulation in nursing education: from conceptualization to evaluation. Washington, DC: National League for Nursing; 2007. p. 42–58.
41. Parsons ME, Hawkins KS, Hercinger M, et al. Improvement in scoring consistency for the Creighton Simulation Evaluation Instrument©. Clin Simul Nurs 2012;8(6): e233–8.
42. American Heart Association. Stroke simulation scenarios. Available at: https://www.stroke.org/-/media/stroke-files/ischemic-stroke-professional-materials/stroke-simulation-scenarios-ucm_500488.pdf?la=en. [Accessed 29 November 2023].
43. Hoh BL, Ko NU, Amin-Hanjani S, et al. 2023 guideline for the management of patients with aneurysmal subarachnoid hemorrhage: a guideline from the American Heart Association/American Stroke Association. Stroke 2023;54:e314–70.
44. The Joint Commission. Standardized performance measures for comprehensive stroke centers. Available at: https://www.jointcommission.org/-/media/tjc/documents/measurement/performance-measurement/measures/stroke/standardized-performance-measures-for-comprehensive-stroke-centers.pdf/. [Accessed 29 November 2023].
45. National Institute of Health. National Institute of Neurological Disorders and Stroke: Stroke Scale. Available at: https://www.ninds.nih.gov/health-information/public-education/know-stroke/health-professionals. [Accessed 29 November 2023].

Use of Simulation for Improving Quality and Patient Safety

Connie M. Lopez, MSN, CNS, CPHRM, CHSE-A, FSSH[a],*,
Kathee Laffoon, MSN/Ed, RN, PHN, RNC-OB, CHSE[b,1],
Jared M. Kutzin, DNP, MS, MPH, RN, FSSH[c]

KEYWORDS

- Healthcare errors • Safety • Quality • Clinical outcomes • Healthcare education
- Healthcare simulation

KEY POINTS

- Simulation can enhance learner outcomes and serve as a mechanism for quality improvement efforts within our complex healthcare organizations and nursing schools.
- Simulation-based education and training offers an immersive and interactive education experience that fosters practice, critical thinking, and confidence in applying knowledge to real-world simulations.
- Simulation can support patient safety and risk management by allowing healthcare teams to identify and address potential safety hazards, practice crisis management scenarios, and develop standardized protocols in controlled, risk-free environments, reducing the likelihood of adverse events in actual patient care settings.

NATURE OF THE PROBLEM AND RECOMMENDATIONS

Healthcare systems continue to look for ways to reduce medical errors, improve patient outcomes, and enhance the quality of care provided. Two years after the sentinel Institute of Medicine (IOM) report highlighting preventable medical errors and the need for efforts at the national level to improve safety, "Crossing the Quality Chasm: A New Health System for the 21st Century"[1] article demonstrated a continued need for improvement centered around safe patient care. The report called for the redesign of healthcare systems to improve the quality of care provided to patients and to

[a] Perinatal Patient Safety, Risk & Patient Safety, Northern California Region, Kaiser Permanente; [b] Center for Learning and Innovation, Scripps Health; [c] Emergency Medicine & Medical Education, Icahn School of Medicine at Mount Sinai, Simulation, Teaching, and Research Center, The Mount Sinai Hospital
[1] Present address: 17412 Plaza Otonal, San Diego, CA 92128.
* Corresponding author. 1800 Harrison Street, 17th Floor, Oakland, CA 94612.
E-mail address: conniemarielpz@yahoo.com

Nurs Clin N Am 59 (2024) 463–477
https://doi.org/10.1016/j.cnur.2024.01.006
nursing.theclinics.com
0029-6465/24/© 2024 Elsevier Inc. All rights reserved.

prevent errors.[2] Within this time, "The Future of Nursing" report[3] recommended changes to the nursing profession to improve healthcare quality and accrediting bodies such as The Joint Commission (TJC), the Centers for Medicare and Medicaid Services, and the National Committee for Quality Assurance set standards for patient care and monitoring to ensure safety and quality. The National League for Nursing also sets education standards for improving the quality of patient care by ensuring nursing students are well-prepared and competent in providing healthcare services. Most recently, TJC published yearly requirements[4] for performing multidisciplinary drills to improve quality patient care and safety.

RESPONSE AND APPLICATION TO RECOMMENDATIONS

The IOM recommended that healthcare organizations promote effective teamwork, communication, and training by utilizing the lessons learned from high-reliability organizations such as the military, aviation, nuclear power plants, and chemical manufacturing trades, all with safety as their highest priority.[5] These complex industries use simulation to explore active and latent safety threats and decrease hazards inherent in these high-risk industries. Applying lessons from these industries to healthcare for training, assessment, research, improving clinical skills, teamwork, and patient safety has reduced medical errors and patient safety[1,6] (**Figs. 1–3**). Healthcare teams practicing for a high-risk event, emergency cesarean section, using simulation in labor and delivery to improve skills, teamwork, and communication.

Simulation can serve as a mechanism for quality improvement efforts within our complex healthcare organizations and nursing schools. It is a teaching methodology that can improve the quality of patient care by allowing healthcare teams to practice and develop clinical skills in a safe and controlled environment. Practicing in a safe environment improves knowledge, competence, confidence, and abilities, improving patient outcomes and providing a more accurate evaluation of clinical skills and decision-making than traditional methods, such as written examinations.[6,7] Providing simulation-based education for students and experienced healthcare teams reduces the risk to actual patients and prevents serious harm by decreasing risk and improving the quality of care. Academic systems have redesigned curriculum from the use of written examinations for assessment to the use of simulation to assess better knowledge application and skills learned. Many healthcare systems have met the challenge of improving the quality of care and patient safety by applying lessons learned from

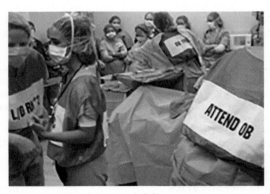

Fig. 1. Emergency cesarean section labor and delivery team.

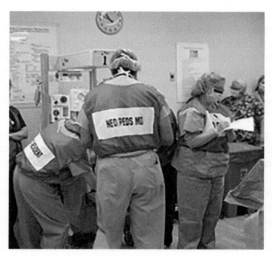

Fig. 2. Emergency cesarean section neonatal team.

highly reliable organizations such as simulation. The following describes how one organization uses simulation to improve quality and patient safety.

Catheter-associated urinary tract infections (CAUTIs) are among the most common hospital-acquired infections, accounting for up to 70% to 80% of adverse outcomes related to indwelling urinary catheter use.[8] Scripps Health, a large, integrated, not-for-profit healthcare organization based in San Diego, California, developed a unique, multipronged approach to reduce CAUTI infections and improve patient safety through education, training, and retraining, standard work with checklists and simulated hands-on training during orientation and annual skills fair. To improve quality and patient safety and reduce the number of CAUTI infections, Scripps formed a multidisciplinary CAUTI Prevention Workgroup to examine the problem, identify gaps and barriers, and produce countermeasures. Through diligent observation, training and

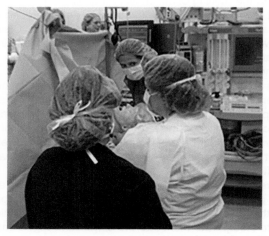

Fig. 3. Emergency cesarean section anesthesia team member with patient and family.

retraining of nurses, and education of staff and physicians, Scripps developed new criteria that reduced the need for catheter insertion, provided alternatives for indwelling catheters, and reduced the length of time for indwelling catheters. Using an evidence-based approach, bedside nurses developed a Standard Work Checklist to be followed by nurses inserting all indwelling urinary catheters. It mandates that two nurses participate in a catheter insertion: One nurse reads each step aloud and monitors the aseptic technique of the second nurse who performs the procedure. The key to the success of this training include.

- Nurses are trained on this standard work during a hands-on simulation and systemwide onboarding orientation. Depending on the unit-specific CAUTI rates, this simulation is repeated during annual skills fair and used individually for retraining.
- Infection prevention staff, risk managers, nurse managers, executives, and front-line staff also monitor the status of CAUTI infection events in real-time using a CAUTI Drilldown Dashboard on their internal intranet site. This dashboard tracks CAUTI data, such as CAUTI events at each hospital, department, and unit, and drivers that increased the risk for each CAUTI event. Examples of the drivers include patient hygiene, standard work followed, and inappropriate indication for catheter insertion and elements that would have helped prevent a CAUTI, such as education, training, retraining, and additional staffing.
- These tools developed and used by bedside nurses have positively impacted patient care satisfaction, quality, and safety.

USING PROCESS IMPROVEMENT TO ORGANIZE PROGRAMS AND IMPROVE QUALITY OF PATIENT CARE

When creating a process improvement educational training program such as the CAUTI program, it is essential to have an organized, systematic approach (**Fig. 4**). All process improvement efforts must have the support and buy-in from leadership. When leadership knows the rationale and elements of the program, they will more likely support the program to ensure success. Involving champions from among critical roles and departments, such as nursing, physicians, executive management, front-line staff, and union leadership, if applicable, will help ensure success as the project evolves and the training commences. All quality improvement efforts should start with the end in mind. Therefore, it is crucial to define organizational outcomes clearly and then narrow this down to learner-specific objectives. Clearly outlining programmatic goals will allow an organization to focus on how the training program will provide a benefit and return on investment (ROI) to their organization. These objectives will drive the agenda of the training program.

Developers of a training program must also understand their learners. Understanding learners' experience level, education, roles, practice area, and setting will determine the next steps after defining goals and objectives. Are learners in an academic setting or acute care setting? Is this an interdisciplinary group of learners, or are they nursing-centric? Would it be advantageous to assess the level of learning with a pre-assessment or pretest before the simulation so that one can compare their learning scores after the educational offering?

Process improvement simulations include various teaching tools such as briefings, pretests, didactic presentations, checklists, and algorithms that augment the simulations. Determine the educational program elements needed to achieve the intended results and plan to incorporate them into the curriculum. **Fig. 4** shows the Develop Curriculum and Teaching Tools. After creating teaching tools, determine the

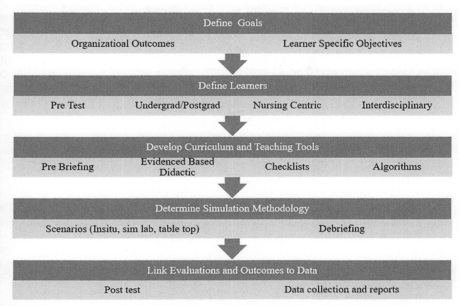

Fig. 4. Process improvement diagram for educational training program template.

simulation methodology and debriefing points. The simulation method can vary based on objectives and include in situ, high/low fidelity, tabletop, or virtual simulation. Focusing debriefing methods on learning objectives is an integral part of performance improvement simulation and measurement for determining program success. Last, all process improvement simulations must include an evaluation and outcome measurement and may be a simple post-test or post-simulation survey of the participants or can include various data collection points and reports to measure ROI and quality improvement indicators linked to organization outcomes. **Fig. 4** outlines a program template. **Fig. 5** applies the template using the CAUTI Reduction Program example.

SIMULATION CONCERNS AND CHALLENGES

Incorporating healthcare simulation into nursing education and ongoing training programs enhances nurses' skills and confidence and contributes to patient safety by reducing error, improving teamwork, and fostering a culture of continuous learning and improvement in healthcare settings. Although a valuable tool, simulation has challenges, including high-cost equipment, training, supplies, and maintenance, which can be prohibitive for healthcare organizations and academic institutions. Depending on the educational objectives and budget, healthcare simulation may involve using simulation technology, including high-fidelity manikins, virtual reality (VR), and standardized patients, to provide more realistic scenarios and environments for healthcare professionals to practice and improve their skills. In addition, faculty require training and education using different simulation and debriefing techniques; this training can be inadequate due to cost, time constraints, and other professional priorities. Finally, students require a high degree of psychological preparation as simulation activities can cause them to be apprehensive and frustrated.[9]

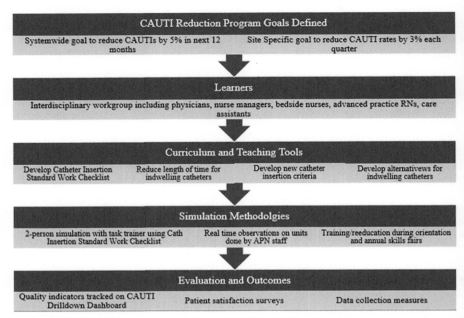

Fig. 5. Process improvement diagram for a CAUTI Reduction Program example.

POTENTIAL SOLUTIONS TO CONCERNS AND CHALLENGES

To mitigate these challenges, educators can use low-fidelity simulators and task trainers, collaborate with other healthcare institutions to share resources, and offer access via remote opportunities such as distance simulation. As a simulation method, distance simulation can potentially to decrease educational costs by allowing students and healthcare professionals to practice skills and procedures without the need for expensive physical equipment or resources. Relatedly, distance simulation can reduce the costs associated with purchasing and maintaining specialized training facilities. Distance simulation enables remote education and training, allows students access to education content, and encourages interaction with instructors from anywhere in the world.[10] In addition, distance simulation has the potential to improve the quality of care through the creation and standardization of curriculum. Instead of relying on varied and potentially outdated educational materials, distance simulation can provide consistent and up-to-date learning modules, reducing costs associated with developing and maintaining educational resources.[10]

Self-guided education and online or eLearning as a form of training are less resource-intensive and can be a wise investment for healthcare organizations needing to decrease their financial burden. In situ and simulation laboratory experiences can augment existing education to meet the needs of various learners and reduce the cost of simulation training. Any practice experience that enhances realism and mimics real-life situations can improve systems thinking and team performance and will increase care quality and patient safety regardless of the mode of simulation training used.

FUTURE INNOVATIVE TOOLS FOR AUGMENTING SIMULATION AND MEETING CURRENT CHALLENGES

VR is one aspect of a broader technology field collectively known as extended reality (XR). XR includes VR, augmented reality (AR), and mixed reality (MR). VR is typically considered a head-worn device that immerses the wearer into an artificial world. AR is typically used with handheld devices that allow the user to see the real world but have specific aspects of AR through digital technology. MR combines VR and AR in that it uses head-worn devices such as a headset or glasses, allowing the wearer to see both the natural world and aspects of the virtual world simultaneously. Each of these technologies can impact patient safety and healthcare quality. Although modern XR technology is still developing, VRs use in medical and nursing education, especially for surgical training has existed for almost 20 years. Evidence demonstrates that the use of VR in training future surgeons leads to improved outcomes both in terms of acquiring skills and "warming up" before entering the operating room.[11,12] Clinically, XR is starting to be used routinely in complex surgeries to allow neurosurgeons and orthopedists (among many others) as opportunity to visualize procedures before conducting them and then overlay specific imagery onto the patient during the procedure.[13] A novel approach using XR during surgery, sold by Microsoft who partnered with a surgeon in New York City, used AR to help a surgeon in Uganda perform a complex procedure with the goal of improving patient care and safety[14] **(Fig. 6)**.

SUPPORT FOR SIMULATION IS NOT NEW: A BUSINESS CASE FOR USE OF SIMULATION

Specialties such as obstetrics and midwifery have been using simulation to improve outcomes for years. For example, to improve maternal safety, a nurse midwife in the eighteenth century in France, Madame du Coudray, designed a homemade task trainer that simulated the childbirth process, allowing her students to practice delivery techniques in a safe and controlled environment.[15] She believed that practicing midwifery techniques on real women was not ideal. Instead, she created the "machine de Coudray" so her students could practice delivering babies and resolving complications, such as shoulder dystocia, without putting the mother and student at risk. Madame du Coudray's innovative use of simulation to teach midwife students improved maternal safety by reducing risks associated with inexperienced practitioners. In addition, it helped elevate midwifery and perinatal nursing by providing a more standardized and systematic approach to childbirth.[15]

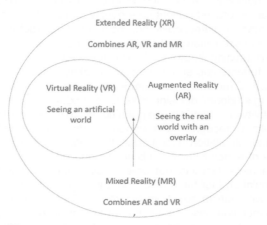

Fig. 6. Extended reality.

Current Need and Evidence for Use of Simulation

Simulation provides valuable opportunities for individuals and teams to practice and hone their collaborative abilities in a safe environment. Using simulation to highlight miscommunication and teamwork issues enhances collaboration and highlights human factors that may be the root cause of potential adverse events.[16] On an individual level, simulation can also improve confidence and competence, making healthcare workers more personally responsible and enhancing readiness. For example, mock codes can prepare providers to respond to emergencies, clarify role expectations, and expose systems issues, primarily when conducted in situ. Simulations performed in situ are a unique opportunity to bring teams together in the actual practice setting using available equipment. During unannounced cardiac arrest simulations performed in situ in the United Kingdom,[1] the 55 team participants agreed that the simulations were an accurate representation of actual cardiac arrest and helpful in training and assessment of both technical and nontechnical skills, improving their performance during patient care.

Simulation has notably improved nursing and medical student education in the following ways.

- Simulation allows students to practice and develop clinical skills in a safe, regulated environment without harming patients. Simulation practice can help improve patient safety by reducing errors, increasing accuracy, and enhancing the quality of care.[17]
- Simulation allows students to gain confidence in their abilities and learn from their mistakes.
- Simulation enables students to encounter various clinical scenarios and patient types, including rare and complex cases in which they may not engage in a clinical setting. Simulated encounters help to broaden students' knowledge and experience base and can help them optimize workflows and reduce errors, resulting in increased efficiency.[18]
- Using simulation to teach interprofessional collaboration and communication skills with team members, patients, and families[19] can reduce misunderstandings, enhance the patient experience, and is essential for providing high-quality, patient-centered care.

Simulation-based education provides a safe and controlled environment for experienced and student nurses to practice and develop skills, improving patient outcomes. Studies demonstrate improved patient care quality and safety for nurses in the pre-licensure, perioperative, pediatric, obstetric, and mental health settings. **Table 1** shows the different studies of simulation applications that impact quality and patient safety.

Simulation-based training improves knowledge, skills, and confidence in pre-licensure nursing students and enhances patient safety outcomes such as reduced medication errors.[19] Simulations also improve communication among obstetric teams[20] and nursing students' decision-making.[21] In addition, education and simulation enhance the ability of pediatric nurse practitioners to manage asthma patients and novice nurses' ability to recognize and respond to deteriorating patients.[22,23] In the perioperative setting, simulation-based education reduces stress and improves the team performance of endovascular scrub nurses and positively affects nursing students' ability to achieve learning outcomes, collaborate, and improve self-confidence.[24] Last, simulation facilitates reflection and experiential learning for students caring for people with autism spectrum disorder.[25] These studies demonstrate the effectiveness of simulation-based education in improving nursing students' knowledge, skills, and confidence and improving patient safety outcomes.

Table 1
Application of simulation to impact quality and patient safety

Audience	Study	Application
Medical residents	Rider and Schertzer,[1] 2022	Procedural simulation resulted in fewer needle passes, arterial punctures, catheter adjustments, and a higher success rate for catheter insertion. Eighty-five percent reductions in procedural-related infections.
Interprofessional stroke team	Rider and Schertzer,[1] 2022	Door-to-needle time decreased from 27 to 13 min.
Midwifery students	Scharf et al,[15] 2022	Designed a homemade task trainer to simulate the birth process, allowing students to practice safe delivery techniques and standardized birthing processes.
Nursing and medical students	Gaba,[17] 2004	Simulation practice can help improve patient safety by reducing errors, increasing accuracy, and enhancing the quality of care. Students gain confidence in their abilities and learn from their mistakes. It enables students to encounter various clinical scenarios and patient types, including rare and complex cases in which they may not engage in a clinical setting.
	Manser,[18] 2009	Simulated encounters help to broaden students' knowledge and experience base and can help them optimize workflows and reduce errors, resulting in increased efficiency.
	Peng Ngo et al,[21] 2023	Improved nursing students' decision-making.
Pre-licensure nursing students	Pol-Castañeda et al,[19] 2022	Simulation-based training has improved knowledge, skills, and confidence and resulted in better patient safety outcomes, better communication with patients, families, and patients, and fewer medication errors.

(*continued on next page*)

Table 1 (continued)		
Audience	**Study**	**Application**
Multidisciplinary obstetric teams	Dillion et al,[20] 2021	Improved communication among obstetric teams.
Pediatric nurse practitioners and novice nurses	Liu et al,[22] 2022; Borgmeyer et al,[23] 2017	Improved ability to manage asthma patients and recognize and respond to deteriorating patients.
Endovascular scrub nurses	Andrea et al,[24] 2022	Reduced stress and improved team performance.
Students caring for people with autism spectrum disorder	Diaz-Agea et al,[25] 2022	Facilitates reflection and experiential learning.

RETURN ON INVESTMENT WHEN SIMULATION IS USED FOR EDUCATION

Quality-based outcomes can be challenging to link to simulation, but examples in the literature demonstrate how simulations have improved patient outcomes, as listed in **Table 1**. For instance, Barsuk and colleagues[26] studied residents who trained using simulation-based medical and education for procedures. Compared with residents who did not receive this training, the simulation-trained residents had fewer needle passes, arterial punctures, catheter adjustments, and a higher success rate for catheter insertion. In another study,[1] more than 32 months, residents trained in the simulation had an 85% reduction in infections compared with those who were not. In addition, researchers conducted multiple in situ sessions with an interprofessional team at their workplace to study door-to-needle time in stroke patients. Following the in situ simulations, they reviewed 650 patients' door-to-needle time and found that critical time decreased from 27 to 13 minutes.[1] These results directly correlate with in situ simulation training and improved patient outcomes.[27]

There is research that examines proficiency-based training programs. In one study,[27] second and third-year residents participated in a 10-hour simulation-based curriculum focused on central venous catheter insertion. Ninety-two residents completed training consisting of lectures, return demonstration, and simulation-based exercises with comprehensive feedback and debriefing. There was a sixfold decrease in catheter-associated bloodstream infections (CABIs) following training compared with the same unit before the training. The cost of this annual training was approximately $112,000 but offset by a net savings of $700,000 from reducing CABI rates.[28] These data show that simulation-based training can save substantial medical costs while improving patient outcomes. Although this research focuses on medical residents, these principles can benefit nurses who insert intravenous and peripherally inserted intravenous central catheter lines. Establishing demonstrated proficiencies is essential for best care practices focusing on patient safety.

SIMULATION RECOMMENDATIONS FROM PROFESSIONAL ORGANIZATIONS AND REGULATORY AGENCIES

The United States ranks 65th among technologically advanced nations regarding maternal death, according to TJC (2019).[4] For the first time, a regulatory agency has published requirements to improve quality of patient care and safety. TJC

Table 2
The joint commission standards for perinatal safety

Maternal Hemorrhage	Severe Hypertension
Simulation Recommendations for Reducing Harm Related to Maternal Hemorrhage	Simulation Recommendations for Reducing Harm Related to Maternal Severe Hypertension/Preeclampsia
Conduct annual multidisciplinary drills to evaluate the hospital's hemorrhage response procedures and perform a post-simulation debrief to determine system issues	Conduct annual multidisciplinary drills to evaluate the hospital's severe hypertension/preeclampsia response procedures and perform a post-simulation debrief to determine system issues

provides accreditation to healthcare facilities in the United States. Alarmed by preventable errors and worsening maternal morbidity and mortality, TJC recently updated its perinatal obstetric hemorrhage and hypertension standards.[4] These standards include the need for regular multidisciplinary simulation drills that focus on system issues to reduce the risk of obstetric hemorrhage and harm related to severe maternal hypertension/preeclampsia (**Table 2**). TJC published yearly requirements[4] for performing multidisciplinary drills to improve maternal care related to postpartum hemorrhage and severe hypertension. For the first time, these perinatal standards emphasize in situ simulations, team debriefs, role-specific education to all staff, providers, and patients, and emergency checklists, crucial for identifying weaknesses in the organization's emergency response system and determining their level of proficiency to improve their quality of care. Tools such as closed-loop communication, root cause analysis, and creating a psychologically safe environment are essential in identifying accomplishments and opportunities for improvement.[4] Using simulation allows healthcare teams to evaluate teamwork, communication, and systems issues that can hinder safe patient care. For the bedside practitioner, these drills result in better training and teamwork, collaboration, and interventions that improve communication.

RESEARCH APPLICATION OF THE JOINT COMMISSION RECOMMENDATIONS AND RESULTS

Team training using simulation improves practitioner skills and teamwork in the obstetric setting decreases patient harm and reduces individual and organizational costs. The Center for Medical Simulation studied a simulation-based team training/crisis management program between 2002 and 2019.[27] They used malpractice claims rates as an outcome to evaluate the efficacy of a medical simulation program within obstetrics. They observed a significant reduction in malpractice claim rates after simulation training and an even more substantial reduction in claims rates if the participant attended more than one session.[27] This study supports the TJC recommendations of yearly simulations and suggests that all team members should participate in multiple sessions to impact harm and claims rates.

Between 2011 and 2013, the National Council of State Boards of Nursing conducted a landmark, national, multi-site, controlled study[29] of replacing clinical hours with simulation in pre-licensure nursing programs across the United States. The first phase of this longitudinal study randomized nursing students to receive varying amounts of simulation instead of traditional clinical experiences, substituting 10% of clinical hours in simulation. Students were placed into three groups.

. The control group with traditional clinical experiences

2. The 25% group, where students replaced 25% of traditional hours with simulation
3. The 50% group, where students had 50% of their clinical hours replaced by simulation

Throughout each core clinical course and each semester, student's clinical competency and nursing knowledge were regularly assessed, and learning needs were evaluated in both the simulation and traditional clinical settings. At the end of their nursing program, there were no statistically significant differences among the three study groups in clinical aptitude, comprehensive nursing knowledge, and the National Council Licensure Examination pass rates. The passing rates of all three groups exceeded the 2013 national average passing rate of 80%.[29] This study provides "substantial evidence that substituting high-quality simulation experiences for up to half of traditional clinical hours produces comparable end-of-program educational outcomes and new graduates ready for clinical practice."[29(pS3)] As a result, hospital administrators, physicians, patients, fellow nurses, and the public can be confident that these newly graduated nurses are competent and knowledgeable regardless of the number of hours spent in clinical training that took place in simulation.

Another group that has provided innovative quality improvement initiatives is the California Maternal Quality Care Collaborative (CMQCC), a multi-stakeholder organization based in California, USA.[30] CMQCC, founded in 2006, dedicates time and resources to improving the quality of maternity care and reducing maternal and neonatal morbidity and mortality. California has seen maternal mortality decline by 65%, whereas the national maternal mortality rate has continued to rise.[30] CMQCC provides evidence-based research and quality improvement resources such as toolkits, simulation scenarios, and checklists to help healthcare providers and facilities implement best practices to improve maternal and infant care. For example, there are at least eight toolkits on various perinatal complications, such as obstetric hemorrhage, hypertensive disorders of pregnancy, maternal sepsis, cardiovascular disease in pregnancy, and the immediate postpartum period. As a result, healthcare organizations can easily access resources such as best practices, care guidelines, checklists, and comprehensive simulation templates at no cost to utilize at the unit level with their direct healthcare providers to improve quality and patient safety.

SUMMARY

Including simulation in healthcare education and training has improved patient safety by helping healthcare professionals identify and address potential sources of errors in both their environments and clinical practice. For example, simulation allows one to practice high-risk procedures, such as emergency resuscitation, in a safe and controlled environment. In addition, practice before an emergency enables healthcare professionals to identify and correct errors in their techniques before treating patients. As demonstrated in the research, simulations used to develop and assess new clinical protocols and procedures can help to reduce the risk of medical errors and improve patient outcomes. When simulation education is introduced early during medical and nurse training, simulation practice can improve patient safety, optimize workflows, reduce medication errors, and teach interprofessional collaboration and communication skills. Finally, by focusing on quality improvement, healthcare simulation can help reduce costs associated with medical errors and improve quality-based outcomes.

Healthcare organizations and academic institutions are addressing recommendations and concerns for safety by incorporating simulation into their educational programs to improve clinical skills, knowledge, and confidence and enhance patient safety by reducing medical errors. Nursing education is focused on a balanced approach combining simulation with traditional clinical experience.

CLINICS CARE POINTS

- Simulation has significantly impacted nursing education and patient safety.
- By providing a safe, controlled environment for students to practice and develop their skills, simulation has improved the quality of nursing education and training.
- Simulation has improved safety and outcomes by helping nursing professionals identify and correct potential sources of error in their practice, resulting in fewer errors and reduced costs.
- Simulation-based training for healthcare teams and nursing students can improve patient safety, optimize workflows, reduce medication errors, and teach interprofessional collaboration and communication skills.

DISCLOSURE

C.M. Lopez: Laerdal Medical Patient Safety Advisory Board Chair, Med VR Scenario Design Consultant. J. Kutzin: Laerdal Medical Patient Safety Advisory Board, Medora Education Scenario Design Consultant, Deputy Editor, Mede Portal (AAMC).

REFERENCES

1. Rider A, Schertzer K. Quality improvement in medical simulation. In: StatPearls. Treasure Island (FL): StatPearls Publishing; 2023. https://www.ncbi.nlm.nih.gov/books/NBK551497/. [Accessed 3 March 2023].
2. Institute of Medicine (US), Committee on Quality of Healthcare in America. In: Crossing the quality Chasm: a new health system for the 21st century323. Washington (DC): National Academies Press (US); 2001. p. 1192.
3. Institute of Medicine. The future of nursing: leading change, advancing health. Washington (DC): National Academies Press (US); 2011. https://doi.org/10.17226/12956.
4. The Joint Commission. R³ Report: PC standards for maternal safety. Provision of care, treatment, and services standards for maternal safety. 2019. https://www.jointcommission.org/-/media/tjc/documents/standards/r3-reports/r3-issue-24-maternal-12-7-2021.pdf. [Accessed 7 May 2023].
5. Guise JM, Segel S. Teamwork in obstetric critical care HHS public access. Best Pract Res Clin Obstet Gynaecol 2008;22(5):937–51.
6. Issenberg SB, McGaghie WC, Petrusa ER, et al. Features and uses of high-fidelity medical simulations that lead to effective learning: A BEME systematic review. Med Teach 2005;27(1):10–28.
7. Bloch SA, Bloch AJ. Simulation training based on observation with minimal participation improves paediatric emergency medicine knowledge, skills, and confidence. Emerg Med J 2015;32(3):195–202.
8. Lo E, Nicolle LE, Coffin SE, et al. Strategies to prevent catheter-associated urinary tract infections in acute care: 2014 Update. Infect Control Hosp Epidemiol 2014;35(5):464–79.
9. Asegid A, Assefa N. Effect of simulation-based teaching on nursing skill performance: a systematic review and meta-analysis. Front Nurs 2021;8(3):193–208.
10. Haerling KA. Cost-utility analysis of virtual and mannequin-based simulation. Simul Healthc 2018;13(1):33–40.

11. Seymour NE, Gallagher AG, Roman SA, et al. Virtual reality training improves operating room performance: results of a randomized, double-blinded study. Ann Surg 2002;236:458–63, discussion: 463–4.

12. Calatayud D, Arora S, Aggarwal R, et al. Warm-up in a virtual reality environment improves performance in the operating room. Ann Surg 2010;251:1181–5.

13. Erickson M. Virtual reality system helps surgeons, reassures patients. Stanford Medicine 2017;. https://medicalgiving.stanford.edu/news/virtual-reality-system-helps-surgeons-reassures-patients.html.

14. Microsoft©. Customer Story: From 7.000 miles apart, Mount Sinai and Ugandan surgeons work together in real time, bringing life-saving expertise to rural communities. https://customers.microsoft.com/en-us/story/f6b7c250-d9b2-4659-8dbf-a44055a8286c?preview=1. [Accessed 1 July 2023].

15. Scharf JL, Bringewatt A, Dracopoulos C, et al. La Machine: obstetric phantoms of Madame Du Coudray , back to the roots. J Med Educ Curric Dev 2022;9. https://doi.org/10.1177/23821205221090168. 23821205221090168.

16. Rudolph JW, Raemer DB, Simon R. Establishing a safe container for learning in simulation. Simul Healthc 2014;9(6):339–49.

17. Gaba DM. The future vision of simulation in healthcare. Qual Saf Healthcare 2004; 13(suppl_1):i2–10.

18. Manser T. Teamwork and patient safety in dynamic domains of healthcare: a review of the literature. Acta Anaesthesiol Scan 2009;53(2):143–51.

19. Pol-Castañeda S, Carrero-Planells A, Moreno-Mulet. Correction: Use of simulation to improve nursing students' medication administration competence: a mixed-method study. BMC Nurs 2022;21(1):154.

20. Dillon SJ, Kleinmann W, Seasely A, et al. How personality affects teamwork: a study in multidisciplinary obstetrical simulation. Am J Obstet Gynecol MFM 2021;3(2):100303.

21. Peng Ngo T, Barnes R, Reising D. Hybrid concept analysis: peer collaborative clinical decision-making in nursing simulation. J Nurs Educ 2023;62(5):269–77.

22. Liu Z, Chen Q, Wu J, et al. Simulation-based training in asthma exacerbation for medical students: effect of prior exposure to simulation training on performance. BMC Med Educ 2022;22(1):223.

23. Borgmeyer A, Gyr PM, Ahmad E, et al. Pediatric nurse practitioners effective in teaching providers the asthma action plan using simulation. J Pediatr Nurs 2017 May-Jun;34:53–7.

24. Andrea R, Lawaetz J, Konge Lars, et al. Simulation-based education of endovascular scrub nurses reduces stress and improves team performance. J Surg Res 2022;280:209–17.

25. Díaz-Agea JL, Macías-Martínez N, Leal-Costa C, et al. What can be improved in learning to care for people with autism? A qualitative study based on clinical nursing simulation. Nurse Educ Pract 2022;65:103488.

26. Barsuk JH, McGaghie WC, Cohen ER, et al. Simulation-based mastery learning reduces complications during central venous catheter insertion in a medical intensive care unit. Crit Care Med 2009;37(10):2697–701.

27. Schaffer AC, Babayan A, Einbinder JS, et al. Association of simulation training with rates of medical malpractice claims among obstetrician-gynecologists. Obstet Gynecol 2021;138(2):246–52.

28. Pacheco Granda FA, Salik I. Simulation training and skill assessment in critical care. In: StatPearls. Treasure Island (FL): StatPearls Publishing; 2022.

29. Hayden JK, Smiley RA, Alexander M, et al. The NCSBN national simulation study; A longitudinal, randomized, controlled study replacing clinical hours with

simulation in prelicensure nursing education. JNR_Simulation_Supplement.pdf. 2014;5(2 Supplement):S1–66. https://www.ncsbn.org/public-files/JNR_ Simulation_Supplement.pdf. [Accessed 1 May 2023].

30. Stanford University School of Medicine. Resources & toolkits. California maternal quality care collaborative. 2022. https://www.cmqcc.org/resources-toolkits. [Accessed 7 April 2023].

Simulation's Use Across the Clinical Landscape

Jared M. Kutzin, DNP, MS, MPH, RN, FSSH, FAAN[a],*,
Connie M. Lopez, MSN, CNS, PHN, CPHRM, CHSE-A, FSSH[b]

KEYWORDS

- Required and specialty certification courses • Nurse onboarding
- Nurse continuing education • Regulatory & joint commission
- Interprofessional education

KEY POINTS

- Many hospitals still have gaps in their use of simulation.
- Simulation is not just useful for knowledge and skill acquisition throughout the clinical environment, but it must also be used as part of a robust patient safety and process improvement program.
- The myriad of uses of simulation requires nursing educators to partner with other sectors of the healthcare team to fully use simulation to affect not only education but also clinical practice and patient care.

INTRODUCTION

Across the healthcare continuum simulation is routinely integrated into the curriculum for nurses and other professionals. The amount of simulation experienced at different points in the clinical setting highly depends on the specialty and organizational investment. Although many healthcare organizations across the United States have invested in simulation equipment and personnel, there is still a gap at many hospitals domestically. Globally the gap is even larger, with developing nations' use of simulation lagging far behind countries with higher gross domestic products.[1] The use of simulation in nursing can be divided into five specific use cases:

Required and Specialty Certification Courses
Nurse Onboarding
Nurse Continuing Education

[a] Emergency Medicine and Medical Education, Icahn School of Medicine at Mount Sinai, Simulation, Teaching, and Research Center, The Mount Sinai Hospital, One Gustave L Levy Place, Box 1149, New York, NY 10029, USA; [b] Risk & Patient Safety, Kaiser Permanente Northern California Region, Oakland, CA, USA
* Corresponding author. One Gustave L Levy Place, Box 1149, New York, NY 10029.
E-mail address: jared.kutzin@mountsinai.org

Nurs Clin N Am 59 (2024) 479–487
https://doi.org/10.1016/j.cnur.2024.02.006
0029-6465/24/© 2024 Elsevier Inc. All rights reserved.

Regulatory & Joint Commission (including annual competencies)
Interprofessional Education

Although common elements exist for each of the abovementioned use cases, there are distinct advantages, disadvantages, and implementation challenges with each that need to be considered.

ELEMENTS COMMON TO ALL SIMULATION

Whenever simulation is being used in the education of nurses, properly trained simulation facilitators must lead or co-lead the program alongside subject matter experts. Using a framework, such as Kern's 6-step model of curriculum development (**Fig. 1**),[2] will help guide the facilitator to ensure that all key elements of the curriculum are considered before implementation. Beginning with the first two steps, general and targeted needs assessment, provides the foundation on which to build or implement the curriculum.[2] Clearly articulating why the curriculum is needed helps direct the educator in how best to use their time and to the best educational methodologies. Writing well-constructed objectives, the third step, is the essential building block for the rest of the curriculum. Using specific, measurable, achievable, relevant, and time-bound (SMART) objectives ensures that the educator and learner can meet the identified needs.[2] Next, choosing the right educational methodology, which may or

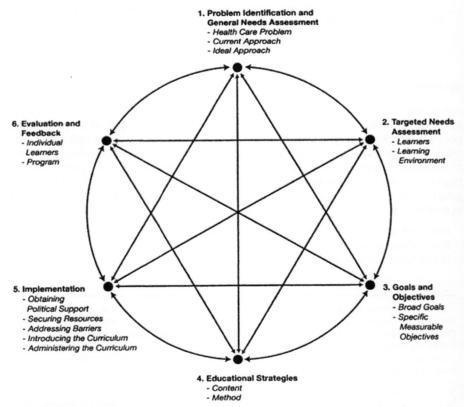

Fig. 1. Kern's 6-step model of curriculum development.

may not be simulation, is the fourth step in the model. The model concludes with the implementation and evaluation of the curriculum.

The fourth step, educational methodology, is where the facilitator has flexibility and creativity in determining the appropriate mode of education. Facilitators may choose to create or provide online content before having learners participate in a simulation. Or facilitators may choose to have learners take part in a simulation that uses a stop-start method of facilitation as opposed to a more traditional simulate-debrief method. Further still, it is at this point in the development process that facilitators may choose a specific type of simulator to use. These may include part-task trainers, high-technology simulators, standardized patients, hybrid simulators, or extended reality devices.[3]

In addition to following a method of curriculum development, nursing professional development educators/professionals must follow standards of best practice put out by organizations like the Society for Simulation in Healthcare and the International Nursing Association of Clinical Simulation and Learning. Many clinical educators are not formally trained in simulation-based education and are ill-prepared to sufficiently use the technique for the education of practicing nurses.

Incorporating simulation into the education of nurses is a rewarding and value-added aspect of many curriculums. Although seemingly costly in the initial upstart, the potential cost-savings and return on investment are significant, but implementation takes forward-thinking leaders committed to excellence.

REQUIRED AND SPECIALTY CERTIFICATION COURSES

Simulation has been the foundation of many required certification programs. The high-technology simulation manikins used today have their base in the 1960s when Drs. Safar, Elam, and Gordon and Norwegian toymaker Åsmund Laerdal collaboratively developed the Resusci-Anne Cardiopulmonary Resuscitation (CPR) manikin.[4] Today, CPR (Basic Life Support), Advanced Cardiac Life Support (ACLS), and Pediatric Advanced Life Support (PALS), among many other courses, use various simulation modalities.

For the better part of 2 decades, CPR researchers have pointed to a degradation of skills after taking the traditional instructor-led training course. As a direct response to the evidence that CPR skills begin to degrade 3 months after training, the American Heart Association and Laerdal Medical introduced a program in 2015 known as RQI (Resuscitation Quality Improvement), which changes the cycle of training from every 2 years to every 3 months.[5] The RQI program introduced a low-dose, high-frequency model of training for clinical staff. Although other training has not yet moved to this model of education, it would seem logical that the more frequently that training is provided, the better.

Other specialty certifications also incorporate simulation into their programs, but the amounts and frequency vary. These certifications include courses such as the Trauma Nursing Core Course and Emergency Nurse Pediatric Course from the Emergency Nurses Association, Advanced Trauma Life Support from the American College of Surgery, Advanced Life Support in Obstetrics from the American Academy of Family Physicians, and PeriOp 101 from the Association of periOperative Registered Nurses, and the American Burn Association.[6]

The benefit of incorporating simulation through these courses is that the potential pushback from administrators and staff regarding cost and time is minimal, because of the required nature of the program. Although the RQI program for BLS, ACLS, and PALS decreases not only staff and facilitator time but also equipment costs, the commitment to hosting the other certification courses and the traditional BLS, ACLS, and PALS programs is significant, requiring the upfront outlay for the purchase of equipment, dedicated space, and educators who are certified instructors.

The downside of introducing simulation through these required courses is that the flexibility and creativity of the facilitators and simulation operations professionals are limited. Because these courses are purchased from national/international organizations, adherence to their requirements is necessary, preventing facilitators from deviating outside the scope of the program; this may lead to participants feeling that the courses are either too advanced or below their current level of achievement and that the course and thereby extension, the simulation, are simply checkboxes they need to fulfill.

The use of simulation has shown remarkable success when implemented as a collaboration between international organizations, such as the American Heart Association, and forward-thinking industry partners, such as Laerdal Medical, who together formed Resuscitation Quality, which follows the best evidence related to both simulation and education. The use of simulation as part of required certifications can add to the experience if implemented in an evidence-based process. The future of simulation in these programs should be guided by the latest research and deployed deliberately for both educators and learners.

NURSE ONBOARDING

Nurse onboarding is fraught with many challenges. These challenges include a lack of educators, a lack of preceptors, a high staff turnover rate, stressful, overcrowded work environments, and a lack of dedicated training space.[7] Evidence demonstrates that onboarding staff is the first step in creating a positive culture and work environment, which in turn results in a commitment to the organization resulting in higher staff and patient satisfaction scores, decreased burnout, and higher staff retention.[5] Nurses leave their positions on the unit for several reasons, including poor leadership, a poor work environment, and career advancement. Simulation, although a powerful tool, cannot be the magic bullet to fix all problems within the healthcare environment. That premise notwithstanding, simulation can be used to help prepare novice nurses for the challenging work environments they encounter in the hospital.[8] The work environment is complicated not only by sicker, more complicated patients but also by the interpersonal interactions that nurses have with each other and the myriad of health professionals they interact with. A variety of simulations can be used to introduce and reinforce teamwork and communication principles during the onboarding period as well as teach and assess clinical knowledge, skills, and attitudes.[7] Evidence has demonstrated that a simulation-based orientation program for nurses has improved knowledge, skills, and attitudes and resulted in decreased onboarding times.[8] However, the amount of such evidence is limited, and recent review articles highlight the need for more research to be conducted on the value of simulation in the onboarding phase.[9] Recent discussions on simulation discussion boards have highlighted the need for hospital-based simulation educators to spend a significant portion of their introductory sessions preparing new nurses for their simulation experiences and establishing a safe container in which to learn because recent nursing graduates arrive with anxiety related to simulation due to poor experiences with the educational technique in nursing school.[10] This "trauma" that nurses arrive with from nursing school related to simulation threatens to undermine the utility of simulation in transitioning new nurses into practice and helping nurses function at their highest level.

Nurse onboarding programs have been developed for many specialty units including the emergency department, intensive care unit, and pediatrics among others. Onboarding programs do not just extend to new registered nurses but also to new Advanced Practice Providers (APPs) entering these units as well. Hospital systems such as the Medical College of Wisconsin, Stanford, and Northwell Health all offer opportunities for APPs to gain in-depth experience in dedicated training programs, which include the use of simulation for skills such as airway management, central line placement, and team leadership.[11–13]

A sample emergency department nurse residency curriculum is included in **Table 1**.

NURSE CONTINUING EDUCATION, REGULATORY REQUIREMENTS, AND INTERPROFESSIONAL EDUCATION

Using simulation in annual competency assessments and for regulatory requirements is an essential component of many simulation programs in the hospital environment. No matter the clinical specialty of the nurse, ensuring they are up to date on the latest

Table 1
A sample emergency department nurse residency curriculum

Session	Objectives	Scenario
1	Complete a focused patient assessment Discover how to use an ED stretcher Review medication administration process Demonstrate oxygen administration process	Asthma • Patient assessment ◦ Signs and Symptoms Allergies Medications Past medical history Last oral intake Events leading up to the current state history ◦ Onset Provocation/palliation Quality Radiation Severity Time history • Oxygen & nebulizer administration Anaphylaxis • Patient assessment ◦ SAMPLE history ◦ OPQRST history • Oxygen, Bag Valve Mask, stretcher operations • Epinephrine, diphenhydramine, Solu-Medrol administration
2	Identify roles during a cardiac arrest Review the use of the defibrillator Discover the process for responding during the "first 5 min" of a code	Rapid cycle deliberate practice of a cardiac arrest[14]
3	Review cardiac arrythmias Implement the correct treatment of brady- and tachy-arrhythmias	EKG review for the novice learner[15]
4	Identify the trauma assessment process Review the treatment of anaphylaxis for a pediatric patient	Traumatic Amputation • ABCDEFGHI trauma assessment • Tourniquet application • Massive transfusion protocol Pediatric Anaphylaxis • Airway management of a pediatric patient • Pediatric assessment triangle • Medication administration for anaphylaxis • Dosage adjustment for pediatric patient

clinical knowledge and required regulatory skills is best achieved through immersive, simulation-based learning. Continuing education can be implemented in a uniprofessional manner or as part of an interprofessional team training experience.[16,17] In obstetrics, research has shown that the self-efficacy of nurses increased after continuing education that used simulation.[10] However, the use of simulation for specific, high-stakes summative assessments in healthcare and in particular nursing is still fraught with challenges.[17] Simulation-based summative assessment requires rigor in the development of objectives, scenarios, and assessment tools as well as competency frameworks and dedicated staff to successfully implement.[18] Although the medical community has long used standardized patients in Objective Structured Clinical Encounters as a form of high-stakes assessment for advancement in the profession, nursing has been slow to adopt standardized patient assessments, especially for continuing professional development. In addition to the rigor needed for summative assessment, learners themselves find the exercise anxiety-producing,[19] which, in turn, may decrease the utility of simulation overall in the clinical environment, as nurses may be reluctant to participate in clinical simulations.

However, the Joint Commission and other regulatory bodies are now requiring health systems to use simulation to improve care processes for patients. The R[3] Report from the Joint Commission discusses Standards for Maternal Safety and Standard PC.06.01.01EP 4 & 5, which encourages in-situ simulations and requires drills annually to assess system issues for patients at risk of presenting with post-partum hemorrhage and maternal hypertension emergencies.[20,21] Although these regulatory requirements focus on system improvements and patient safety, clinical providers may often feel as if they are the ones being assessed, and care must be taken to keep the focus of these assessments on the system and not on individual provider knowledge or skill.

The regulatory drills and other system-focused simulations often focus on the interplay between providers, departments, and the system of care. The purpose is to find opportunities to improve teamwork and communication and discover how human factors may affect care.[22] Including TeamSTEPPS-related concepts of teamwork, communication, situation monitoring, and role clarity into the simulation objectives results in teams functioning at their highest levels in systems that support high-quality, safe care.[23]

The use of simulation in nursing continuing professional development should be expanded. However, the time commitment needed to include simulation for the entire nursing population in a healthcare setting is a significant challenge. Although simulation provides an improved learning environment, it often necessitates smaller groups, which in turn results in extended time to engage the entire learner population. When nurses, physicians, and other health professional staff learn with, from, and about one another in a simulated setting they are exposed to the realistic work environment in which they may operate. Identifying each other's roles and strengths only improves the opportunity to provide the best care to patients. However, interprofessional education likely further reduces the number of nurse learners participating in a particular simulation as the other professions must also be accounted for.

When developing a continuing professional development program, educators must decide if the specific knowledge, skills, and attitudes that need to be obtained, certified, or validated are solely aimed at the nursing staff, in which case expanding the number of learners but keeping it uniprofessional would be ideal, or whether the goal is to identify and improve the team dynamics in which case a smaller number of nursing participants involved in an interprofessional simulation would be better. Either way, the role of high-quality simulation cannot be overstated. It has the power to engage, change, and validate nursing professionals across the continuum.

SUMMARY

Simulation has become a common educational technique in nursing school. However, nurses in clinical practice may be reluctant to fully embrace simulation due to poor experiences in previous educational environments, a fear of being assessed, or poorly constructed simulation education programs by unprepared nursing professional development educators in the clinical environment. Following standards of best practice and guidelines provided by professional societies and further developing their professional practice to include robust education on simulation education are methods that nursing professional development educators can use to improve their use of simulation education. Simulation is not just useful for knowledge and skill acquisition throughout the clinical environment, but it must also be used as part of a robust patient safety and process improvement program. This myriad of uses of simulation requires nursing educators to partner with other sectors of the healthcare team to fully use simulation to affect not only education but also clinical practice and patient care.

CLINICS CARE POINTS

- Standardized simulation programs are available from specialty societies that use simulation in varying amounts and intensities.
- Simulation can be used for knowledge and skill acquisition but should also be used for system-based improvements in care.
- Regulatory bodies are beginning to encourage the use of in-situ simulation in an effort to improve healthcare safety and quality.

REFERENCES

1. Sawyer T, Gray MM, Umoren R. The global healthcare simulation economy: a scoping review. Cureus 2022;14(2):e22629.
2. Thomas PA, Kern DE, Hughes MT, et al. Curriculum development for medical education: a six-step approach. Baltimore, MD: Johns Hopkins University Press; 2015.
3. Lioce L, Lopreiato J, Founding Ed, Downing D, Chang TP, Robertson JM, Anderson M, Diaz DA, Spain AE, the Terminology and Concepts Working Group. In: Healthcare simulation dictionary. 2nd Edition. Rockville, MD: Agency for Healthcare Research and Quality; 2020. https://doi.org/10.23970/simulationv2. AHRQ Publication No. 20-0019.
4. Tjomsland N. Saving more lives - together. The vision for 2020. Laerdal Medical Corporation; 2015.
5. Cheng A, Nadkarni VM, Mancini MB, et al, American Heart Association Education Science Investigators; and on behalf of the American Heart Association Education Science and Programs Committee, Council on Cardiopulmonary, Critical Care, Perioperative and Resuscitation; Council on Cardiovascular and Stroke Nursing; and Council on Quality of Care and Outcomes Research. & American Heart Association Education Science Investigators; and on behalf of the American Heart Association Education Science and Programs Committee, Council on Cardiopulmonary, Critical Care, Perioperative and Resuscitation; Council on Cardiovascular and Stroke Nursing; and Council on Quality of Care and Outcomes Research. Resuscitation Education Science: Educational Strategies to

Improve Outcomes From Cardiac Arrest: A Scientific Statement From the American Heart Association. Circulation 2018;138(6):e82–122.

6. Carrougher G, Burton-Williams K, Gauthier K, et al. Burn Nurse Competency Utilization: Report From the 2019 Annual American Burn Association Meeting. J Burn Care Res 2020;41(Issue 1):41–7.

7. Kurnat-Thoma E, Ganger M, Peterson K, et al. Reducing Annual Hospital and Registered Nurse Staff Turnover—A 10-Element Onboarding Program Intervention. SAGE Open Nursing 2017;3. https://doi.org/10.1177/2377960817697712.

8. Pena H, Kester K, Cadavero A, et al. Implementation of an Evidence-Based Onboarding Program to Optimize Efficiency and Care Delivery in an Intensive Care Unit. Journal for Nurses in Professional Development 2023;39(6):E190–5.

9. Pogue DT, O'Keefe M. The Effect of Simulation-Enhanced Orientation on Graduate Nurses: An Integrative Review. J Cont Educ Nurs 2021;52(3):150–6.

10. Kardong-Edgren S, Wells-Beede E. Stop Prelicensure Student Abuse in Simulation. SimZine. 2023. Available at: https://simzine.news/focus-en/sim-nurse-en/stop-prelicensure-student-abuse-in-simulation/. [Accessed 1 December 2023].

11. (n.d.). MCW. Advanced Practice Providers. Medical College of Wisconsin. 2024. Available at: https://www.mcw.edu/departments/mcw-advanced-practice-providers/app-fellowship-np-residency-programsaccessed.

12. (n.d.). APP Fellowship Program. Stanford medicine health care 2024. Available at: https://stanfordhealthcare.org/health-care-professionals/nursing/departments/center-for-advanced-practice/app-fellowship-program.htmlaccessedJanuary28.

13. (n.d.). Advanced Clinical Provider Fellowship. Northwell Health. Available at: https://2022-acp-fellowship.ttcportals.com/. [Accessed 28 January 2024].

14. Kutzin JM, Janicke P. Incorporating Rapid Cycle Deliberate Practice Into Nursing Staff Continuing Professional Development. J Cont Educ Nurs 2015;46(7):299–301.

15. Kutzin J, Milligan Z, Justiniano S. EKG Review for the Novice Learner. MedEdPORTAL 2014;10:9952.

16. Ehmke S, Swan M, Van Gelderen S, et al. Impact of obstetric emergency high-fidelity simulation on maternity nurses' self-efficacy in the rural hospital setting. American Journal of Maternal/Child Nursing 2021;46(3):150–4.

17. Keddington A, Moore J. Simulation as a method of competency assessment among health care providers: a systematic review. Nurs Educ Perspect 2019; 40(2):91–4.

18. Buléon C, Mattatia L, Minehart RD, et al. Simulation-based summative assessment in healthcare: an overview of key principles for practice. Adv Simul 2022; 7:42.

19. Arrogante O, González-Romero GM, López-Torre EM, et al. Comparing formative and summative simulation-based assessment in undergraduate nursing students: nursing competency acquisition and clinical simulation satisfaction. BMC Nurs 2021;20:92.

20. American College of Obstetricians and Gynecologists. "Preparing for Clinical Emergencies in Obstetrics and Gynecology." ACOG Committee Opinion No. 590. Obstet Gynecol 2014;123:722–5.

21. The Joint Commission. R³ Report: Requirement, Rationale, Reference. Provision of Care, Treatment, and Services standards for maternal safety. Issue 2019;24.

22. LeBlanc VR, Manser T, Weinger MB, et al. The study of factors affecting human and systems performance in healthcare using simulation. Journal of the Society for Simulation in Healthcare 2011;6(Suppl):S24–9.

23. King HB, Battles J, Baker DP, et al. TeamSTEPPS™: Team Strategies and Tools to Enhance Performance and Patient Safety. In: Henriksen K, Battles JB, Keyes MA, et al, editors. Advances in patient safety: new directions and alternative approaches. Rockville (MD): Agency for Healthcare Research and Quality (US); 2008. Performance and Tools. Available at: https://www.ncbi.nlm.nih.gov/books/NBK43686/.

Simulation for Competency Development in Clinical Practice

Catherine Morse, RN, PhD, AGACNP-Ret, CHSE[a],*,
Sabrina Beroz, DNP, RN, ANEF, CHSE-A[b],
Mary K. Fey, PhD, RN, CHSE-A, ANEF[c,1]

KEYWORDS

- Simulation ● SimZones ● Competency

KEY POINTS

- Competency is not a static concept and needs to be reinforced and reassessed.
- Skill decay affects competency and needs to be included in the educational plan.
- Using a shared language and process of competency in education and practice has the potential to reduce the education–practice gap.

INTRODUCTION

A competent nurse or nurse practitioner is the goal for academic and professional providers. However, the collective profession has struggled to implement consistent terminology, incorporate evidence-based teaching practices and close the education–practice gap. It is not an uncommon refrain to disparage the preparation of our new colleagues as not being prepared for real life in clinical practice. It is the aspiration on both sides—education and practice to have competent graduates. Competency-based education (CBE) is now on the front burner of nursing education at the undergraduate and graduate levels with the proposal from the American Association Colleges of Nursing 2021 Essentials with the intent to transform nursing education curricula and to close the education-to-practice gap.[1] This proposed transformational change in how we educate has the potential to influence professional education and to tackle the long-standing education–practice gap. The education–practice or theory–practice gap

a College of Nursing and Health Professions, Drexel University, Health Sciences Building, 8th floor CICSP, 60 North 36th Street, Philadelphia, PA 191104, USA; b Montgomery College, National League for Nursing, 812 Crystal Court, Gaithersburg, MD 20878, USA; c Center for Medical Simulation, Boston, MA, USA
1 Present address: 1606 Grange Road, Edgewater, MD 21037.
* Corresponding author.
E-mail address: cjm69@drexel.edu

Nurs Clin N Am 59 (2024) 489–498
https://doi.org/10.1016/j.cnur.2024.01.010
0029-6465/24/© 2024 Elsevier Inc. All rights are reserved, including those for text and data mining, AI training, and similar technologies.
nursing.theclinics.com

has been described in the literature for many years as the gap between the assessment of a successfully graduate registered nurse (RN) exiting an academic program and the same RN entering practice.[2,3] Simply put, it is the differences between "what should happen" and "what does happen" or put another way, work as imagined and work as done. This gap is continually evolving as nursing practice, technology, and healthcare advances have dramatically changed over the decades.

Zieber and Wojtowicz (2019) proposed that we stop thinking of theory and practice as separate realities and that we can dwell in both spaces on a continuum.[2] This idea is critical as we think about simulation and competency across the spectrum of pre-licensure education, professional practice, and the new graduate advanced practice nurse (APN). The tightening of this relationship has important potential impacts to ease the transition to practice for new graduates of all levels (new to practice and advanced practice), to positively impact patient safety and new graduate retention in the profession. We are proposing that using the same language and principles across fundamental education and professional practice using CBE and simulation is the right vehicle for this partnership.

This article will explore the relationship between CBE and simulation, to close the education–practice gap for new graduate nurses or new APNs transitioning to practice and maintaining clinical competency. SimZones will be used as an example of a curricular planning and design tool.[4]

BACKGROUND

A desire to improve patient safety is driving the focus on clinician competence in healthcare and health professions education. CBE was first used in the 1960s to support the training and development of elementary school teachers.[5] Recently, more higher education programs are implementing CBE, especially in the health professions.[1,6–10] The defining feature of CBE that sets it apart from traditional time-based educational frameworks is a focus on the end products of education, that is, what the learner can do, as opposed to the inputs of education or training programs, that is, the content of lectures and readings, or number of hours spent.[1,8–10] As graduates come to practice with experience and knowledge of competency-based learning and evaluation, they will push the practice side to continue to evolve. This grass-roots culture change has the potential for positive change.

Additional features of CBE include a focus on outcomes, deemphasis on time-based training, the promotion of learner-centeredness, more formative assessment, and direct observation of learners' skills and abilities with frequent feedback.[6,7] The "one-and-done" approach to testing a skill does not ensure competence because competence is context-dependent and demonstrates the integration of knowledge, skills, ability, and judgment.[10] The American Nurses Association describes competency as an ongoing process, not a one-time outcome.[11]

Simulation provides a method for both developing and assessing competence. See **Box 1** for key concepts of CBE.

Simulation-based education and CBE aligns with the learners born after 1982. This generation of learners expects experiential learning, frequent feedback, interactions with their peers, and likes to feel a sense of accomplishment from their work. These expectations are met by simulation and CBE.[5] Simulation allows for the construction of different contexts in which to develop and assess competence. New to practice nurses and APNs can experience varied settings (eg, in patient, outpatient, and home care) with a variety of patients (eg, different ages, genders, ethnicities, levels of acuity, diagnoses, and comorbidities). Their clinical training experiences will be

---

Box 1
Key concepts of competency-based education

Competence is not a static concept

It is learner-centered not instructor-driven

Formative assessment: Assessment and feedback for learning is frequent

Competence looks different depending on our expertise (A competent novice nurse looks different than a competent expert nurse)

Simulation can be used to develop and evaluate competence at all levels of expertise

---

varied and prepared them as a generalist for the new graduate nurse and for their chosen specialty as an APN. As they come to clinical practice, simulation-based education can provide the level playing field allowing for multiple specialties, varied clinical settings, and increasing complexity (**Box 2**). Clinicians, new to practice and experienced, can first be taught an isolated skill, and then be challenged to demonstrate that skill in various realistic contexts (eg, low-stress "routine" call, higher stress emergency situation, and in conversation with someone who speaks a different native language). The SimZones curricular framework supports this scaffolded process with strong consideration given to the learners being "ready" to be in the learning space.[4,12,13]

Simulation can, and should, be used for both formative and summative assessment. For the purposes of this discussion, summative assessment is competency assessment or demonstration, whereas formative assessments are made in the service of learning. During formative learning experiences, the instructor provides support and coaching as scaffolding that lessens over time. Initially, with acquisition of a new skill (including psychomotor and relational), formative experiences require specific instruction and helpful coaching as the learner encounters the desirable difficulties of learning. As the learners' skill develops, less-directive coaching is required, and the instructor becomes more of a facilitator of reflective learning to help the learner discover personal challenges that may be standing in the way of skill development.[12] Formative learning experiences should occur prior to competency assessment, and the assumption of being taught in lecture translating to skill acquisition should be challenged because knowledge does not automatically translate to doing. The number and frequency of formative learning opportunities will vary based on the experience of the learners, the complexity of the skill, and frequency at which the skill is practiced in patient care. See **Fig. 1** as an illustration of the relationship between requisite knowledge, formative assessment, and competency (summative) assessment.

Traditionally most new graduates engage in a new graduate residency program that can vary in length and process, then transition to the assigned clinical role and

---

Box 2
Key characteristics of current new graduates

Familiar and expects experiential learning

Wants frequent developmental feedback

Enjoys working with peer groups

Enjoys a sense of meaning or accomplishment from work

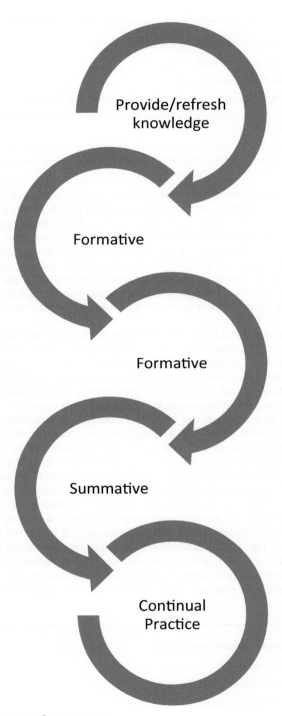

Fig. 1. Iterative process of competence.

specialty followed by an annual competency evaluation of skills defined by the clinical unit and specialty. This process does not consider skill decay and other factors such as cognitive load. Skill decay refers to the concept that if not used, skill competency fades in weeks to months. Research demonstrates that skill decay can vary depending on the expertise of the learner, the complexity of the skill, and relevance to the learner.[14,15] Considering skill decay into the development of competency programs is critically important because demonstrating a skill or clinical thinking annually for high-risk, low-frequency events does not maintain competency for when the skill is needed in clinical practice. This concept challenges the assumption that annual competency evaluation confers continued competence for the rest of the year irrespective of the frequency at which the skill is performed.

Simulation-based education can be used in the formative and summative stages of the competency journey. In the formative phases, it allows participants to be practicing the skills (psychomotor or cognitive) in a similar environment with a similar cognitive load paired with reinforcing and developmental feedback. Reinforcing feedback expands on positive performance and assists the learners to make connections to different clinical situations. Developmental feedback assists the learners to close the gap between performance and the agreed upon standard of care. The competency standards or behaviors are transparently shared with the learners prior to the formative phases, and it is the same standard of assessment that is used in the summative competency assessment.

Simulation provides a mechanism by which summative assessments can be standardized across learners. Summative assessment experiences, especially any that affect a person's employment or advancement in a program, demand the highest level of rigor. This rigor includes the simulation case, learner preparation, and assessor training. Facilitators, assessors, and simulated patients (if using) should be trained in the principles of simulation and evaluation techniques; evaluation instruments must show evidence of validity and reliability; learners must have had multiple exposures to formative simulations prior to summative assessment; and learners must be adequately oriented to the assessment process and the environment.[16] Simulation cases should be peer reviewed by content experts and tested prior to use with the learners.[17]

Patient safety is a value shared across professions in healthcare. Simulation affords a unique opportunity to train clinicians for competence across levels of expertise and practice settings. It also provides a mechanism to safeguard patient safety by evaluating that competence. It is incumbent for the educator to be transparent about the level of assessment—formative or summative. An ongoing program of simulation for formative and summative assessment can be an important strategy or organizational improvement. Implementing this type of curriculum can seem daunting at first and using a supportive framework can make the work more accessible. The next section of the article will introduce SimZones as a curricular framework.[4,12,13]

SimZones

The SimZones curricular framework supports competency development in healthcare.[4,12,13] Building an integrated curriculum that supports clinician competence in the complex skills currently required for clinical practice requires careful sequencing and consideration. In the SimZones framework describes learning in 4 zones as clinicians develop expertise.

Zone 0: Learners acquire or refresh the prerequisite knowledge for the skill. It often includes automated devices or computer programs that provide feedback to the learner. The instructor's role in Zone 0 is as the designer and not of immediate feedback giver.

Examples include cardiopulmonary resuscitation (CPR) manikins with automated feedback, or an online escape room with expert feedback at predetermined decision points.

Zone 1: It is instruction in the foundational skills, which may be psychomotor, communication, or teamwork skills. Learners are instructed and practice the skill without a clinical context (eg, role play in a classroom and intubating on a manikin head/airway). Instructors provide expert feedback and coaching in the moment.

Zone 2: Those new skills are further developed in a realistic clinical context in Zone 2 simulations. For example, simulation-based education may be a pause and discuss scaffolded approach with a manikin-based case.

Zone 3: It is for ongoing development of individuals or teams. An interprofessional team caring for the same type of patient in Zone 2; here the scaffolds are pulled back and learners work to solve the clinical case in a realistic context and engage in a reflective debriefing. The primary role of the instructor is as facilitator.

Zone 4: It is learning from real-world practice (eg, debriefing actual clinical events).

A WORKED EXAMPLE

As a nurse educator, you are working in an academic medical center and have the responsibility over the new nurse residency program. The unit council has identified the concern that new nurse residents are not comfortable caring for patients with acute respiratory distress and desaturations. There have been multiple rapid response calls and unplanned transfers to the intensive care unit. The nurse residents in their weekly reflective debriefs have also identified they are not feeling comfortable with noticing and responding to changes in patient condition in this population.

Identified learning needs: Nurse residents are perceived to not be competent in identifying patients in respiratory distress, choosing the most appropriate oxygen delivery device, and giving an urgent situation background assessment and recommendations (SBAR) handoff to other team members in an urgent situation.[18] Through shared discussions, the key knowledge and skills were defined by the learners and educator. Content expertise was sought from the pulmonary service nurse practitioner. See **Table 1** for the summary of identified knowledges and skills.

The proposed zone-based learning would be as follows:

- Zone 0: The learner independently reviews oxygen delivery devices which may include matching exercises with patient condition and choice of device in the online learning space, and the nursing monitoring and documentation required. The

Table 1 Knowledge and skills summary: caring for a patient with respiratory distress	
Knowledge	**Skills**
Normal and abnormal vital signs	Conducting a focused physical examination
Early and late signs of respiratory distress	Conducting a focused history
Oxygen delivery devices available	Identification of abnormal findings
Indications for starting oxygen	Setting up and running common oxygen devices
Hospital policies	SBAR communication with rapid response team (RRT) team
Components of SBAR	Patient positioning
How and when to access rapid response	

components of SBAR are reviewed and the nurse identifies incomplete and complete SBAR from viewing simulated hand-offs. This is completed independently with automated feedback. This could take the form of online matching, hot spot identification with automated feedback, watching short videos with follow-up questions and expert feedback.

- Zone 1: The learner works with an instructor to learn to demonstrate what focused assessments to complete and correctly apply and/or operate the different types of devices in a skills laboratory setting. This could include moving from the simple (nasal cannula to the complex, noninvasive positive pressure ventilation). The skill practice is conducted without clinical context. Typically, this would occur in a skills laboratory with appropriate equipment. The learner would also demonstrate SBAR handoff given different clinical presentations. The instructor would provide coaching and instructions as needed.
- Zone 2: The learner now encounters a simulated patient in respiratory distress and demonstrates clinical assessment and decision-making about what device to apply, when to collaborate with other members of the healthcare team, and when a true respiratory emergency is at hand requiring a rapid response or medical emergency response team. This is still a scaffolded learning setting, and this can be achieved with a pause and discuss approach or having an embedded coach in the simulation.
- Zone 3: An interprofessional team now cares for the simulated patient in a realistic context and practices a team-based approach to managing the respiratory distress requiring oxygen support. The learners demonstrate all the knowledge and skills previously identified and practiced in this setting. Here the team will complete the care of the patient and then participate in a reflective debriefing.
- Zone 4: This is not a simulation but rather ongoing team learning in the real world. For example, a clinical debrief following a real respiratory emergency on the ward where the team works to learn from real-life experiences.

SCENARIO DEVELOPMENT TO SUPPORT COMPETENCY-BASED EDUCATION

Designing cases to support Zones 2 and 3 learning needs to be evidence based and the Healthcare Simulation Standard of Best Practice Simulation Design (2021) states simulation-based experiences (SBE) are purposely designed to meet defined objectives and expected outcomes.[16] Before the simulation can be developed, a needs assessment should be conducted to outline the problem. **Box 3** summarizes key needs assessment questions to be addressed.

Once these questions are answered, the educator can begin to design the learning experience based on the learners' needs and aligning the facilitative approach across the SimZone framework to build competence. Prior to the design of the simulation cases in Zones 2 and 3, it is critical to ascertain that the learners are "ready" to be

---

Box 3
Key needs assessment questions

What recent events led to the need for education?

Who are the internal and external stakeholders?

What are the competencies to be learned and assessed?

What are the learner priorities?

What are the learner outcomes?

Table 2
Design considerations across the zones

SimZone	Learning Goals	Modality	Team	Signal/Noise	Feedback/Debrief
0	Demonstrate Types and uses of oxygen devices Standards of care Components of SBAR	No instructor Virtual simulation or online modules	No team	Clear focus on content (oxygenation) and clinical handoff No noise (distraction)	Automated feedback, expert feedback in writing, or video
1	Demonstrate foundational skill: Types and uses of oxygen devices Clinical documentation SBAR handoff	Instructor-guided learning Deliberate practice	Individual or partial team	Clear focus (signal) Minor noise (distraction)	Instructor feedback, coaching, and teaching
2	Demonstrate Assessment of a patient in respiratory distress Application of correct O$_2$ delivery device for a patient in respiratory distress SBAR handoff to team members	Instructor facilitated: Simulator-based in simulation center or in-situ	Partial or full teams	Increased complexity (signal) Significant noise such as monitors or human interactions	Instructor feedback, coaching and teaching combined with facilitation when needed Pause and discuss approach or postsimulation debriefing with a theory-based model: Coaching (and teaching if needed)
3	Team and system development Demonstrate appropriate assessment and care of a patient severe respiratory distress	Full-scale interprofessional simulation	Full team	Competing clinical indicators and significant noise (complicating care management)	Facilitated debriefing postsimulation

n that Zone and have refreshed and practiced the identified skills that will then be practiced in context in Zones 2 and 3. A competency assessment can be completed at the end of Zone 1 before moving to a Zone 2 simulation.

This staged approach where teaching and learning is aligned across a trajectory of learning from foundational skills to mastery of skills in realistic context to team-based experiences.[12] There is a developmental relationship between the learner and context for learning. When designing learning experiences, the SimZones framework provides the faculty with a sturcture to ensure the learners have the requisite knowledge and skill to be in the intended simulation exercise. For example, a mismatch occurs when the learner is placed in a SimZone 3 simulation without prerequisite knowledge to build competence along a continuum of learning.

Other elements for consideration is simulation design across the zones including the concept of signal and noise, the uniprofession versus team learners, type of learning modality, and feedback/debriefing plan. Signals are desired clinical data or cues and noise is interruptions or distractions that hinder attention to important information.[4] Modality refers to type of learning process, and feedback/debriefing describes the deliberate process of reflection and feedback. **Table 2** provides a worked example or these concepts across Zones using the earlier example described in the article.

SUMMARY

As nursing education transforms to incorporate CBE into the curriculum, this presents an opportunity to close the education–practice gap utilizing simulation as the teaching tool. Simulation is uniquely positioned to provide formative and summative learning experiences for the new to practice nurse or nurse practitioner and to maintain competency for the currently practicing professional. Using a common curricular design tool, such as SimZones, creates consistency of language and learning design for the learners and eases transition into practice. Integrating simulation as both the formative and summative assessment tool will require hospital-based educators to gain and maintain competency as simulation-based educators to leverage this tool. Challenging our long-held practices of annual competency assessments without planned skill decay prevention will be an important step to improving nurse/APN competencies and patient safety.

DISCLOSURE

Dr C. Morse has no commercial or financial conflicts of interest to report. There are no funding sources to report; Dr S. Beroz has no commercial or financial conflicts of interest to report. There are no funding sources to report; Dr M.K. Fey has no commercial or financial conflicts of interest to report. There are no funding sources to report.

REFERENCES

1. American Association of Colleges of Nursing. The Essentials: Core competencies for professional nursing education. 2021. Available at: https://www.aacnnursing. org/Portals/0/PDFs/Publications/Essentials-2021.pdf. [Accessed 15 November 2024].
2. Zieber M, Wojotowicz B. To dwell within: Bridging the theory-practice gap. Nurs Philos 2020. https://doi.org/10.1111/nup.12296.
3. Kalogirou MR, Chauvet C, Yonge O. Including administrators in curricular redesign: How the academic-practice relationship can bridge the practice-theory gap. J Nurs Manag 2020;29:635–41.

4. Roussin CJ, Weinstock P. SimZones: an organizational innovation for simulation programs and centers. Acad Med 2017;92(8):1114–20.
5. Nodine TR. How did we get here? A brief history of competency-based higher education in the United States. J Competency-Based Edu 2016;1(1):5–11.
6. Desy JR, Reed DA, Wolanskyj AP. Milestones and Millennials: A Perfect Pairing-Competency-Based Medical Education and the Learning Preferences of Generation Y. Mayo Clin Proc 2017;92(2):243–50.
7. Frank JR, Snell LS, Cate OT, et al. Competency-based medical education: theory to practice. Med Teach 2010;32(8):638–45.
8. Vasquez JA, Marcotte K, Gruppen LD. The parallel evolution of competency-based education in medical and higher education. The Journal of Competency-Based Education 2021;6(2):e1234.
9. Kavanagh JM, Sharpnack P. Crisis in Competency: A Defining Moment in Nursing Education. Online J Issues Nurs 2021;26(1).
10. Altmiller G. Curriculum Mapping for Competency-Based Education: Collecting Objective Data. Nurse Educat 2023;(5). https://doi.org/10.1097/NNE.0000000000001462.
11. American Nurse Association Position statement: Professional Role Competence. American Nurses Association. Available at: https://www.nursingworld.org/practice-policy/nursing-excellence/official-position-statements.
12. Fey MK, Roussin CJ, Rudolph JW, et al. Teaching, coaching, or debriefing With Good Judgment: a roadmap for implementing "With Good Judgment" across the SimZones. Advances in Simulation 2022;7(1):1–9.
13. Roussin C, Sawyer TWeinstock P, Weinstock P. Assessing competency using simulation: the SimZones approach. BMJ Simulation & Technology Enhanced Learning 2020;6(5):262.
14. Stanley B, Burton T, Percival H, et al. Skill decay following Basic Life Support training: a systematic review protocol. BMJ Open 2021;11:e051959.
15. Offiah G, Ekpotu LP, Murphy S, et al. Evaluation of medical student retention of clinical skills following simulation training. BMC Med Educ 2019;19:263.
16. INACSL Standards Committee. Healthcare Simulation Standards of Best PracticeTM Evaluation of Learning and Performance. Clinical Simulation in Nursing 2021. https://doi.org/10.1016/j.ecns.2021.08.016.
17. INASCL Standards Committee. Healthcare Simulation Standards of Best Practice™Simulation Design. Clinical Simulation in Nursing 2021. https://doi.org/10.1016/j.ecns.2021.08.009.
18. Agency for Healthcare Research and Quality. Tool: SBAR. Available at: https://www.ahrq.gov/teamstepsprogram/curriculum/communication/tools/sbar.html. [Accessed 26 November 2024].

The Role of Simulation in Graduate Nursing Education
Preparing Learners for Practice

Tracie White, DNP, ACNP-BC, CRNFA, CNOR, CHSE[a],*,
Becky Suttle, DNP, BS, CRNP, AGACNP-BC[b],
Tedra Smith, DNP, CPNP-PC, CNE, CHSE[c]

KEYWORDS

• Advanced practice • Simulation • Education

KEY POINTS

• There is a need for providers in the healthcare system.
• Graduate nursing education plays a pivotal role in shaping the future of healthcare by preparing advanced practice nurses.
• Simulation-based education is an effective approach to bridge the gap between theory and practice.

INTRODUCTION

There is an increasing need for providers in the healthcare system, and advanced practice nurses (APRNs) are positioned to help meet those needs. Graduate nursing education plays a pivotal role in shaping the future of healthcare by preparing advanced practice nurses to provide high-quality patient care and to meet the evolving demands of the healthcare system. However, a lack of clinical sites, willing preceptors, and qualified nursing faculty hinders the ability to prepare learners to meet these demands.[1] Nursing education programs are tasked with preparing graduates who possess not only a strong theoretic foundation but also the practical skills and clinical judgment necessary to safely function in a complex healthcare system. Simulation-based education (SBE) is an innovative and effective approach to bridge the gap between theory and practice, offering a controlled and immersive environment for learners to develop clinical competency.[1]

[a] The University of Alabama at Birmingham School of Nursing, 1701 University Boulevard, Birmingham, AL 35294, USA; [b] The University of Alabama at Birmingham School of Nursing, 1720 2nd Avenue South NB 428D, Birmingham, AL 35294-1210, USA; [c] The University of Alabama at Birmingham School of Nursing, 1720 2nd Avenue South, NB 406, Birmingham, AL 35294-1210, USA
* Corresponding author.
E-mail address: twhite220@uab.edu

Nurs Clin N Am 59 (2024) 499–510
https://doi.org/10.1016/j.cnur.2024.02.005
0029-6465/24/© 2024 Elsevier Inc. All rights reserved.
nursing.theclinics.com

SBE has emerged as a powerful tool in graduate nursing education by recreating real-world clinical scenarios in a risk-free environment.[2] It uses various modalities, virtual reality, standardized patients, and technological resources to replicate situations and procedures. The benefits of simulation in graduate nursing education are multifaceted and include skill acquisition, decision-making, team collaboration, navigating difficult conversations, and improving patient safety. The effectiveness of simulation to reduce the theory-practice gap in graduate nursing education is supported by an extensive body of research, and numerous studies have demonstrated improved learner outcomes in such areas as clinical competence, confidence, and preparedness for practice.[3]

This paper explores various types of SBE available for graduate nursing programs and provides examples of graduate nursing simulations that educators can use in their own programs to prepare clinicians for practice.

BACKGROUND

Simulation scenarios encompass a wide array of situations, from simple procedures to complex high-stakes trauma resuscitation.[4] These scenarios are carefully designed to reflect real clinical situations, and they can be repeated until the learner feels confident in their abilities. The complexity of simulated clinical scenarios can be increased to mimic real patient situations as learners progress in their programs.[5] As a result, learners graduate with not only theoretic knowledge but also practical proficiency, thus ensuring their readiness for clinical practice. Simulation is not confined to traditional nursing skills alone. It extends to ethical dilemmas, cultural sensitivity, communication, and other essential relationship skills that are equally vital for providing holistic patient care.[4]

ESSENTIALS AND COMPETENCIES

The American Association of Colleges in Nursing (AACN) provides the framework for academic nursing programs at colleges and universities with their Essentials series. The latest version, "The Essentials: Core Competencies for Professional Nursing Education," was published in 2021 and supports the use of simulation in advanced level nursing education. The AACN notes that simulation provides a safe environment for learning and demonstrating competency and can augment direct clinical care; however, it stops short of allowing simulation to replace direct patient care. Instead, the AACN allows for national specialty organizations and national certification and regulatory agencies to determine if this is appropriate for the specialty. With the move toward competency-based education, simulation takes a key role in advanced nursing education, as it allows learners to repetitively practice high-risk and/or low-frequency experiences. The AACN encourages programs to use simulation best practice standards as outlined by the International Nursing Association for Clinical Simulation and Learning (INACSL) or the Society for Simulation in Healthcare.

The National Association of Nurse Practitioner Faculties (NONPF), the AACN, as well as many other nursing organizations and certification boards formed the National Taskforce on Quality Nurse Practitioner Education (NTF). The NTF updated their standards in 2022 to include a criterion on simulation. Criterion III.K supports simulation in nurse practitioner (NP) education, but simulation hours do not count as direct patient care hours (NTF Standards, 2022). The NTF supports simulations designed to meet competency and follows outlined best practices for development such as INACSL.

EVALUATION OF LEARNING

Formative assessment fosters personal assessment by providing constructive feedback and developing strategies to progress toward the outlined objectives.[6] Learning is the overall goal with formative assessment. The intent is to create an environment that facilitates learning and the development of competencies.[7] Formative assessment provides a chance for reflection on specific outcomes and monitoring progress.

Summative assessment is used to evaluate learning at the end of a program or conclusion of a particular subject. In simulation, summative assessment often focuses on specific outcomes that relate to specific objectives.[6] Learners should be told they will be evaluated for a grade before the simulation. Simulation experiences conducted for a summative assessment should occur after learning a particular concept to assess competence. It is imperative that the facilitators are trained in the principles of simulation and have appropriate, validated evaluation tools.[7]

High-stakes evaluation may be used to assess competence or identify gaps in knowledge or patient safety concerns.[7] High-stakes evaluations are used to determine pass or fail with significant consequences for the learner. One example is the objective structured clinical examination (OSCE) often used to assess clinical competence in advanced practice nursing. The OSCE has long been used to ensure a fair and equitable method to evaluate competence in advanced assessment.[8] When conducting a high-stakes evaluation, facilitators should use a simulation experience that has been implemented previously, the evaluation tool should be validated and use more than one trained observer if it is an observer-based tool, and the experience should be based on specific learner objectives.[7] SBE can be used to achieve goals in all of these situations.

FIDELITY AND MODALITY IN SIMULATION

SBE involves creating a realistic environment to facilitate learning and skill development. Fidelity in simulation refers to the degree of realism in replicating real-world context. Aspects of fidelity include physical, conceptual, psychological, functional, and sociologic.[9] Physical fidelity explains how the learner senses the environment around them (smell, sight, touch, etc.). Conceptual realism refers to a clinical scenario being as close to real as possible as far as how the case presents and unfolds. Psychological fidelity concerns the emotional reaction of the simulation participants, and functional fidelity concerns the precision and realism of the psychomotor skills used during the simulation.[9] Sociologic realism refers to the interactions among interprofessional simulation participants. Each aspect of fidelity has elements that could facilitate or impede the simulation.[9]

SBE also uses various types of modalities that can increase fidelity to provide a realistic and immersive learning experience. These modalities include manikins, standardized patients, and task trainers.[6] The INACSL Standards of Best Practice encourage realism to promote achievement of the established learning outcomes.[6] It is important to remember that simulation does not require high-fidelity methods to be effective and educators should be careful to avoid unnecessary cognitive burden on learners participating in simulation as well as consider resource-allocation when designing resource-heavy simulation.[9] Several exemplars follow demonstrating how different fidelity and modality types can be used in graduate nursing education as well as to maintain skills as a healthcare provider after graduation.

APPLICATION EXEMPLARS
High-Fidelity

Several different modalities of simulation can be used together or separately to achieve high-fidelity simulation. High-fidelity manikins can be combined with other modalities to create a high level of realism for more experienced learners.[9] This example expands on how high-fidelity simulation can be used in advanced practice nursing education.

Exemplar I: Neonatal nurse practitioner transition to practice simulation

Using high-fidelity manikins, learners participated in a final transition-to-practice simulation that centered on prioritization (**Fig. 1**). This program is a distance-based program and brings learners to campus in their final semester. The simulation includes the management of several neonatal patients with various conditions within a realistic neonatal intensive care unit environment. The simulation area included a four-room unit with a nurse's station in the middle. On one side of the unit was a private room (room 1) with a term baby experiencing opioid withdrawal (mother in the room) and room 2 with two patients: a term baby with hypoglycemia and a 26-week-old preemie requiring endotracheal intubation, total parental nutrition, and lipids. Rooms 3 and 4 held the same patient cases. The fifth room was the simulated operating room (OR), which held an emergent neonatal resuscitation case. Two learners could take part in the simulation at one time (one on each side of the unit) with embedded simulation participants calling an NNP learner to the OR at alternating times for the coding patient. The day before the simulation learners were provided with a list of assigned patients and given their patients' charts for review. They were given more patients than appeared in the simulation. This mimics the process of learning about your patients before taking the assignment. To increase realism, actors played the mother at the bedside, hospital administration faculty simulated rounds, a simulated EMR was used for diagnostic and laboratory results, and respiratory therapy was available for patient care.[10]

Exemplar II: AGACNP readiness for practice simulation

This example describes how high-fidelity simulation was used for a readiness for practice simulation for an adult-gerontology acute care NP program that focused on assessment, diagnosis, and creating a treatment plan. This program is a distance-based program that brings learners to campus during the first semester of clinical training for formative simulation focused on diagnosis and treatment. During this simulation learners performed a full patient visit with one patient in an emergency room setting. The patient was a high-fidelity manikin with faculty providing the voice of the patient (**Fig. 2**). The patient complained of shortness of breath and the learner was asked to perform a focused physical assessment, order, and review diagnostics (laboratory results, electrocardiogram, and chest

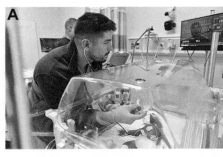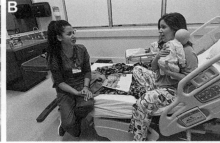

Fig. 1. (*A*) Neonatal transition to practice simulation with high-fidelity manikin. (*B*) Neonatal transition to practice simulation with standardized patient and manikin. (Image Courtesy: UAB School of Nursing/Frank Couch.)

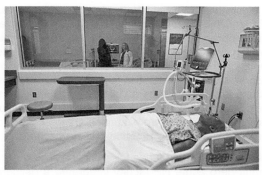

Fig. 2. High-fidelity manikin for AGACNP readiness to practice. (Image Courtesy: UAB School of Nursing/Frank Couch.)

X ray), and then create a treatment plan. An embedded participant acted as a staff nurse and supplied diagnostics upon request. The correct diagnosis was a pleural effusion, and the plan should have included placement of a chest tube for drainage. At the end of the simulation, the learners were led to a debriefing room and then taken to a skills room with task trainer stations set up for practicing chest tube placement. A faculty member staffed the skills room and gave real-time coaching and feedback about the procedure, which learners had already learned about the prior semester but had not yet practiced.

Standardized Patients

The use of standardized patients (SPs) in graduate (or advanced level) nursing simulation creates opportunities for nurse educators to simulate clinical experiences in a safe environment. SPs are volunteers or hired actors trained to portray real patients with specific healthcare issues based on the simulation.[11] The training may include emotional behaviors, communication style, specific body movements to mimic symptoms, and other behaviors as indicated by the scenario.

Simulation experiences with SPs provide the most realistic opportunity to further develop clinical decision-making skills and merge academia with clinical.[12]

Exemplar: Giving bad news
In this simulation, an SP assumed the role of a patient receiving pathology results that confirm the presence of cancer. Learners were tasked with communicating these findings with professionalism and empathy while using an evidence-based framework to guide their discussion. In this scenario, the use of a trained SP was crucial as they conveyed real emotion using facial expressions, voice, and body language. The simulation would not be as effective using a manikin.

Task Trainers

Task trainers are specialized models designed for learners to practice specific skills.[13] In advanced practice training, task trainers are often used for teaching, practicing, and validating procedural skills that require repetition and refinement before performing on a live patient.

These are often considered high-risk skills or procedures that could be painful for the patient, such as central venous line insertion or endotracheal intubation. Task trainers can range in fidelity and cost. They can be used alone for procedural simulation or can be integrated into more complex simulations such as hybrid simulation or an OSCE.

Although scope of practice can vary from state to state for advanced practice nurses, the AACN Essentials support the role of the NP to independently perform clinical procedures when appropriate, and the NONPF NP competencies make specific suggestions as to which procedures should be considered for inclusion in NP curriculum based on population. Training in these procedures is included in advanced practice educational programs with opportunities for learners to show basic competency. Programs often require learners to pass a validation of these skills before allowing them to perform the skills with their preceptor during a clinical rotation. This validation is typically done using task trainers. Two examples are described to expand on how task trainers can be used in advanced practice nursing education.

Exemplar I: AGACNP deliberate practice for skills acquisition

In this activity, adult-gero acute NP faculty integrated a deliberate practice (DP) teaching-learning method into an on campus procedural skills assessment using task trainers. In this program, procedural skills must be assessed to ensure basic competency as learners enter clinical rotations. Task trainers are a key component to this validation, however as many NP programs are distance-based or online, learners often have limited or no interaction with the task trainers prior to coming to campus for the high-stakes evaluation.

Learners received procedural videos with rubrics detailing the expected steps and outcomes for each skill via their online learning platform 4 weeks before the on-campus activity. Reviewing the videos and rubrics beforehand provided a foundational understanding of each skill. At their on-campus intensive four essential procedural skills were practiced and assessed using a DP method (thoracentesis, central venous line, intubation, and lumbar puncture). Skill stations were arranged in a large classroom and staffed by AGACNP program faculty. Teams of five learners moved through each station together.

Using task trainers and rubrics, faculty facilitated repetitive practice cycles. Pre-planned pauses breaking each procedure into smaller portions allowed for deliberate practice which included real-time self-reflection, peer feedback, and faculty coaching. Pausing and starting again from a certain point or from the beginning, allowed learners to master the most difficult steps of the procedure before moving on. After about an hour and several repetitions, learners completed the procedure from start to finish for individual assessment before moving to the next station (**Fig. 3**). These skills can be added to subsequent simulations involving higher level decision making as learners progress in the program.

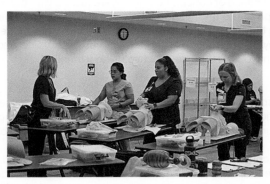

Fig. 3. AGACNP students practicing intubation with task trainers. (Image Courtesy: UAB School of Nursing/Frank Couch.)

Exemplar II: Registered Nurse First Assistant difficult case simulation
Learners enrolled in the Registered Nurse First Assistant (RNFA) subspecialty used
task trainers to practice surgical skills, teamwork, and decision-making. In this
example, the RNFA learners in a distance-based program report to campus for
skills practice before their clinical rotation. During one of the on-campus sessions
learners use the Simulab's Universal Surgical Abdomen Training System while
participating in a simulated case in the OR (**Fig. 4**). This high-fidelity task trainer
is used to provide learners with a realistic and immersive experience in abdom-
inal surgery. Learners were supplied with the necessary surgical instruments, su-
tures, surgical drapes, and other necessary surgical items. The abdomen model
replicates anatomic structures and was connected to a system that simulates
bleeding and suction. Each learner was assigned a specific role within the surgical team (surgeon or assistant). During the case, an unexpected complication
occurred, and learners had to collaborate and communicate effectively to ensure
smooth workflow and patient safety.

HYBRID

Hybrid simulations are designed for several types of scenarios but often work best for
scenarios that incorporate assessment of a psychomotor skill. Hybrid simulation is
defined as the merging of two or more modalities to create a realistic experience for
learners. Merging of modalities allows nurse educators to blend different concepts
into one experience. Two examples are described to expound on how to design
and implement a hybrid simulation.

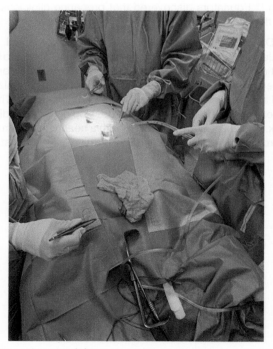

Fig. 4. RNFA students using Simulab's Universal Surgical Abdomen Training System. (Image
Courtesy: UAB School of Nursing/Frank Couch.)

Exemplar I: Pediatric disaster simulation

This exemplar allowed pediatric acute care NP learners to experience providing care after a disaster. Learners were in their final course of the program. The scenario included a bus carrying a multigenerational group on a field trip that was involved in an accident. The neighboring hospital had accepted as many patients as they could, but all others were directed to the pediatric facility (the simulation area at the school of nursing). Patients included children and adults of various ages (**Fig. 5**). The simulation incorporated SPs, low-fidelity and high-fidelity manikins, and task trainers. The scenario began with the NPs being called to the emergency department to help with a mass causality. Learners were left to disperse themselves into teams to care for patients in five examination rooms, one in the hallway on a stretcher and a pregnant woman currently in pain. The patients in rooms were SPs with task trainer injuries such as lacerations. As the simulation progressed, additional SPs acting as parents looking for their children entered the simulated area (**Fig. 6**).

DISTANCE SIMULATION

The COVID-19 pandemic highlighted the need for distance-based activities at all levels of education. The simulation community embraced this challenge, creating a variety of simulation experiences that could be delivered via various platforms, such as Zoom, to learners all over the world. There is a myriad of different potential combinations that can fall under the umbrella of distance simulation. For example, the learners, facilitators, and simulation operators each can be local or distanced relative to one another or relative to a defined location or they can include asynchronous versus synchronous learning.[14] Educators discovered that preparing clinicians for practice did not only occur in the simulation laboratory.

- *Exemplar I*: DNP (Doctor of Nursing Practice) project proposal

This exemplar describes a creative way to prepare DNP learners to present a quality improvement (QI) project plan. The intent of the experience is for learners to present the project idea to key stakeholders of a simulated organization for buy-in, support, and alignment with organizational outcomes needs. This simulation allowed DNP learners to practice planning, developing, and leading QI initiatives, critically think, and collaborate effectively with a healthcare team. It was delivered via Zoom, providing a convenient and innovative way for distance-accessible

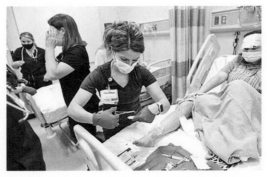

Fig. 5. Hybrid simulation with standardized patient and task trainer leg. (Image Courtesy: UAB School of Nursing/Frank Couch.)

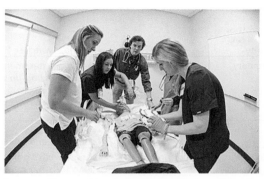

Fig. 6. Hybrid simulation with manikin and standardized patient. (Image Courtesy: UAB School of Nursing/Frank Couch.)

learners to get feedback before presenting their QI projects to stakeholders in the clinical setting. Expectations for the experience were provided within the course along with guidance for preparing the presentation, participant requirements, organization of the virtual event, and the post-event evaluation rubric.

Learners prepared a 12-slide presentation with team and topic introductions, description of the initiative site and participants, identification of a process gap, evidence, proposed process change, stakeholders and workforce, timeline, financial considerations, and sustainability.

A structured faculty–developed prebrief video was placed in the course 1 week before the event. This prebrief video followed the Healthcare Standards of Best Practices: prebriefing and added statements addressing distance simulation elements such as using a camera, signing in with real names, and dealing with technical issues.[15,16] Learners were required to watch the video before the simulation event. On the day of the simulation, each team logged in via Zoom, and the event coordinator gave a prebrief reviewing objectives, fiction contract, basic assumption, and repeated instructions for help with technical issues. The event coordinator then placed learners into virtual breakout rooms where the EPs were waiting in the role of Director of Quality Improvement. Learners shared their screens and presented the project proposal (20 minutes) followed by a 5-minute question session by the EPs. Following the presentation, the learners were moved to the debriefing breakout room.

- *Exemplar II*: CNL (Clinical Nurse Leader) simulation

For this distance-based simulation experience, two scenarios were developed that engaged the CNL learners in the leadership role and fostered intraprofessional communication among nursing leadership and staff. Two simulation-based experiences occurred during the final semester of the CNL program. During the first simulation, video vignettes of a nursing assistant and a nurse caring for and placing an indwelling urinary catheter were placed into the course. CNL learners watched the videos and made notes about potential improvements that were needed. For the second simulation, charts from a virtual EMR were placed in the course. Learners performed a chart review of six patients who experienced a pressure injury. They were to find patterns that could explain why these patients had the injury. After forming a plan for each scenario, the CNL learners met via Zoom to present the data and plan to ESPs in the role of nursing leadership and staff.[17]

Table 1		
I-PASS communication tool		
I	Illness severity	• Stable, "watcher," unstable
P	Patient summary	• Summary statement • Events leading up to admission • Hospital course • Ongoing assessment • Plan
A	Action list	• To do list • Time line and ownership
S	Situation awareness and contingency planning	• Know what's going on • Plan for what might happen
S	Synthesis by receiver	• Receiver summarizes what was heard • Asks questions • Restates key action/to do items

• *Exemplar III*: I-PASS asynchronous simulation

Transition of care is a crucial time when patient safety is vulnerable. It is important that smooth and safe transitions are made when providers hand-off patients to each other.

Very few learners report seeing formal hand-off processes used in their own clinical rotation setting. I-PASS (**Table 1**) is one tool that can be used to aid in teaching provider hand-off processes. For this assignment, learners completed required reading about transitions of care and then watched a video on how the I-PASS tool was developed and how it can be used in practice. Learners identified a patient from their own NP clinical rotation and practiced handing-off this patient to an oncoming provider. They recorded a short video in Go React using the I-PASS framework (initial posts include the "I-PAS" portions of I-PASS). Then learners had 1 week to choose two of their classmates' posts to respond to via recorded video—this is the last "S" in I-PASS and stands for synthesis. In completing the last "S," learners closed the communication loop and practiced a safe patient hand-off. NP students often do not get to participate in the patient hand-off at the end of a clinical day, and many providers do not use a formal hand-off tool. This assignment allowed the learners to practice a safe hand-off using a validated and widely accepted tool. Because this is a distance-based program, it was important to be able to practice this skill in an asynchronous way, and Go React is a tool that allows that to be done, while supporting classmate interaction.

SUMMARY

Simulation in graduate nursing education can significantly translate to clinical practice after graduation. Using the exemplars discussed earlier as well as others, simulation can achieve many goals including the following:

• Skill acquisition: simulation allows learners to practice and refine their clinical skills in a controlled environment. These skills, such as taking vitals, administering medication, wound care, and communication techniques, directly apply to real-world nursing practice.
• Confidence building: through simulation, learners gain confidence in their abilities to handle various scenarios they might encounter in clinical settings. This confidence

carries over into their professional practice, enabling them to approach patient care with more assurance.

- Decision-making skills: simulations often present learners with scenarios that require critical thinking and decision-making. These skills are crucial in clinical practice, where nurses must make rapid and accurate decisions in patient care.
- Familiarity with equipment and technology: simulation exposes learners to a variety of medical equipment and technology used in healthcare settings, such as the electronic medical record. This familiarity helps them adapt quickly to similar tools during their professional practice.
- Teamwork and communication: SBE often involves teamwork and communication exercises, which are essential in clinical practice. Nurses must effectively communicate with patients, families, and other healthcare professionals, and simulation helps develop these skills by placing learners in situations where communication is the goal.
- Emotional preparedness: simulations can also expose learners to emotionally challenging situations, but this occurs in a place where psychological safety is prioritized. Working through these situations helps them understand and manage their emotions when faced with similar situations in real clinical settings.
- Adaptability: through exposure to different scenarios in simulation, learners manage adapting to changing circumstances. This adaptability is crucial in healthcare, where situations can evolve rapidly.

This article aimed to describe the effectiveness of simulation in graduate nursing education and provides exemplars for practical application. The incorporation of simulation into advanced practice nursing education has increased significantly over the past few years. Most advanced practice nursing education programs are distance accessible with limited face-to-face classroom interaction. Simulation has provided a means to assess competence in psychomotor skills and affective and cognitive skills such as delegation, communication, and problem solving.[4] Simulation bridges the gap between knowledge and application, and the various modalities afford nurse educators with the ability to design creative simulations to meet learner needs as they prepare for safe clinical practice. Although simulations cannot replicate every aspect of real clinical practice, they provide a solid foundation for learners. They offer a bridge between theory and real-world application, allowing graduates to enter the workforce with a level of preparedness and confidence that might otherwise take longer to develop solely through traditional classroom learning.

CLINICS CARE POINTS

- Simulation-based education can and should be used to prepare advanced practice nurses for clinical practice.
- Using the appropriate type of equipment (task trainer, high-fidelity manikin, standardized patient) increases realism in a scenario to mimic the clinical setting.
- Simulation-based education is appropriate for practicing clinicians to maintain and improve both clinical skills and team communication.

DISCLOSURE

Dr T. White has no commercial or financial conflicts of interest to report. There are no funding sources to report. Dr B. Suttle has no commercial or financial conflicts of interest to report. There are no funding sources to report. Dr T. Smith has no commercial or financial conflicts of interest to report. There are no funding sources to report.

REFERENCES

1. Hussein M, Osuji J. Bridging the theory-practice dichotomy in nursing: The role of the nurse educators. J Nurs Educ Pract 2016;7(3):20–5.
2. Seaton P, Levett-Jones T, Cant R, et al. Exploring the extent to which simulation-based education addresses contemporary patient safety priorities: A scoping review. Collegian 2016;26(1):194–203.
3. Brown J. Graduate nurses' perception of the effect of simulation on reducing the theory- practice gap. SAGE Open Nursing 2019;5:1–11.
4. Nye C, Campbell SH, Hebert SH, et al. Simulation in advanced practice nursing programs: A North American survey. Clinical Simulation in Nursing 2019;26:3–10
5. Cant RP, Cooper SJ. Simulation-based learning in nurse education: Systematic review. J Adv Nurs 2010;66(1):3–15.
6. INACSL Standards Committee. Healthcare Simulation Standards of Best PracticeTM Evaluation of Learning and Performance. Clinical Simulation in Nursing 2016;58:14–21.
7. McMahon E, Jimenez F, Lawrence K, et al. Healthcare Simulation Standards of Best Practice™ evaluation of learning and performance. Clinical Simulation in Nursing 2021;58:54–6.
8. Hickey M. Objective structured clinical examinations as a method of competency evaluation in a primary care nurse practitioner program. Nurse Educat 2021; 46(5):317–21.
9. Carey JM, Rossler K. The how when why of high fidelity simulation. In: StatPearls [Internet]. Treasure Island (FL): StatPearls Publishing; 2023. Available at: https://www.ncbi.nlm.nih.gov/books/NBK559313/.
10. Wood T, Dudding K, Littleton C, et al. Transition to practice simulation: interprofessional Engagement to Build realism. Birmingham, Alabama: Poster presented at: *UAB Center for* Interprofessional Education and Simulation's 3rd Annual Interprofessional Healthcare Symposium: Building Inclusive Environments Within Interprofessional Teams; 2021.
11. Goodman J, Winter S. Review of use of standardized patients in psychiatric nursing education. J Am Psychiatr Nurses Assoc 2017;23(5):360–74.
12. Barber LA, Schuessler JB. Standardized patient simulation for a graduate nursing program. J Nurse Pract 2018;14(1):e5–11.
13. Singh M, Restivo A. Task trainers in procedural skills acquisition in medical simulation. In: StatPearls [Internet]. Treasure Island (FL): StatPearls Publishing; 2023 Available at: https://www.ncbi.nlm.nih.gov/books/NBK558925/.
14. Duff J, Kardong-Edgren S, Chang TP, et al. Closing the gap: a call for a common blueprint for remote distance telesimulation. BMJ Simulation & Technology Enhanced Learning 2021;7(4):185–7.
15. INACSL Standards Committee. Healthcare Simulation Standards of Best Practice™ Evaluation of Learning and Performance. Clinical Simulation in Nursing 2021;58:14–21, 54-56.
16. McDermott D, Ludlow J. A prebriefing guide for online, virtual, or distant simulation experiences. Clinical Simulation in Nursing 2022;67:1–5.
17. Ledlow JH, Layton SS, Dailey KD. Immersing clinical nurse leader students into the leadership role using remote simulation-based learning experiences. Presented at: CNL Summit, Leveraging CNLs in a Time of Change; 2021. virtual.

Moving?

Make sure your subscription moves with you!

To notify us of your new address, find your **Clinics Account Number** (located on your mailing label above your name), and contact customer service at:

Email: journalscustomerservice-usa@elsevier.com

800-654-2452 (subscribers in the U.S. & Canada)
314-447-8871 (subscribers outside of the U.S. & Canada)

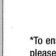

Fax number: 314-447-8029

Elsevier Health Sciences Division
Subscription Customer Service
3251 Riverport Lane
Maryland Heights, MO 63043

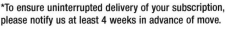

*To ensure uninterrupted delivery of your subscription, please notify us at least 4 weeks in advance of move.

Printed and bound by CPI Group (UK) Ltd, Croydon, CR0 4YY

08/05/2025

01864748-0009